DISCOVER
AYURVEDA

DISCOVER
AYURVEDA

ANGELA HOPE-MURRAY
TONY PICKUP

Ulysses Press Berkeley, CA
1998

Published by: Ulysses Press
P.O. Box 3440
Berkeley, CA 94703-3440

Library of Congress Catalog Card Number: 97-61010

ISBN: 1-56975-081-5

Printed in Canada by Best Book Manufacturers

First published as *Healing with Ayurveda*, Gill & Macmillan, 1996

10 9 8 7 6 5 4 3 2 1

Editorial: Lily Chou
Typesetter: David Wells
Cover Design: B & L Design
Indexer: Sayre Van Young

Distributed in the United States by Publishers Group West and in Canada by Raincoast Books

ACKNOWLEDGEMENTS

*With thanks to the teachers: Dr. Vasant Lad and
Dr. Robert Svoboda; for many hours of help: Laura Miles.*

TABLE OF CONTENTS

WHAT IS AYURVEDA?

Ayurveda means "the science of life." An ancient Indian medical system, it is holistic in the true sense of the word in that it gives priority to the involvement of the patient in his or her own well-being.

Ayurveda empowers you to take control of your own health and life with the aim of preventing illness, as opposed to only treating disease once it has arisen. For example, if you have a headache you will be recommended a treatment and also be asked to look at the imbalance in your lifestyle, environment, diet and mind that has elicited the pain. Once the imbalance is identified, there are short-term traditional remedies that are frequently helpful. More importantly, long-term treatments will enable you to live in such a way that the cause of the pain will not return.

PERFECTION

We all seek the peace associated with perfect health of mind, body and spirit and would love to achieve perfect bliss (if we believe that this is feasible). Life is like a set of scales: it is possible, by using the appropriate measure of each of life's ingredients, for perfect balance to be achieved and illness to disappear. This balance is an integration of body, mind and spirit, leading ultimately to perfect bliss.

THE ELEMENTS

Health may be defined as perfect balance between body, mind, spirit and the environment. The basic tenet of Ayurveda is that the body is composed of the elements earth, air, fire, water and ether. Our bodies are made up of combinations of these elements (as is the food we eat or anything else we come into contact with). Intake of, or contact with a particular element will tend to increase that element within ourselves; therefore, eating a chili will cause a sensation of heat because it is a fiery food. This also applies to our thoughts and the effect that they have on our physical bodies: we are what we think. Everything entering the body — heat, thoughts and experiences as well as food — must be first digested or else it will be incorporated into our being in an unsuitable form that will cause disease. Similarly, excesses or deficiencies in our diet, environment or thoughts that the digestive process cannot compensate for lead to excesses or deficiencies of particular elements in our bodies, creating imbalance and hence disease.

IMBALANCE AND ILLNESS

The aim of Ayurveda is to avoid excesses in life (food or otherwise) and to supplement what is deficient. Importantly, what may be sufficient for one person may be deficient or excessive for another, depending upon his or her basic constitution. All diseases are seen as caused by imbalance, an imbalance that can be resolved by achieving balance in whatever the patient is suffering from, be it a headache, depression, anxiety, insomnia, arthritis or asthma. As well as restoring balance, it is important that the actual cause of the imbalance is removed on an ongoing basis by appropriate attention to diet and lifestyle. For example, there are some herbs that can help create balance or restore correct functioning in the alimentary canal where food digestion takes place. The healthy intestine also regulates what is absorbed from the food we eat and is thus effective in maintaining balance.

In this book we will describe the various elemental forces acting in the mind and body and how they give rise to imbalance and illness. We will also explain how they can function together in health. This book will empower you to change your life for the better and remove those annoying ailments we all tend to put up with. If you are thinking about visiting an ayurvedic practitioner we will tell you what to do before you go, what to expect once you get there and what it all means.

Today, the principles and practice of ayurvedic medicine are being increasingly employed by many, not only in India but also in Europe, Australasia and North America, as part of a holistic approach not just to disease, but to all aspects of everyday life.

THE HISTORY
OF AYURVEDA

The origin of Ayurveda can be traced to ancient times. The story in the *Charaka Samhita*, one of the oldest ayurvedic medical texts, reads like this. Fifty of the most eminent sages gathered together on the slopes of the Himalayas to discuss how to get rid of the common diseases that were causing so much ill health among human beings and interfering in the performance of their duties. They came to the conclusion that Indra, Lord of the Immortals, should be sought out since he knew Ayurveda, or the science of life. He was supposed to have learned this from the physicians of the gods. They, in turn, had learned their knowledge from Brahma, the Creator. Sage Bharadvaya volunteered to go to Indra, who shared his knowledge. It proved most effective.

Many other versions abound and are similar to stories in other cultures; just as Brahma explained Ayurveda to the Indians, Apollo and Thoth revealed the Greek and Egyptian systems of medicine to their respective peoples.

THE ORIGINS OF AYURVEDA

Let us now look at the "facts" as far as they are known. It is difficult to be precise about the start of civilization in India and about the historical origins of Ayurveda since all dates are unrecorded prior to the time of Buddha (563-483 B.C.). The earliest civilizations appear to have been the Harappa, which existed in the Indus Valley from circa 3000 B.C. until 1500 B.C. They were a successful race and achieved a society similar to the one created in Rome much later. There is very little evidence of a medical system although one must have existed. It was probably the Aryans, a group of people from the Caucasus, invading and mixing their systems with those of the Harappa, who introduced Ayurveda.

The Aryans brought with them a new body of wisdom and religious practice and probably took on some of the local Harappan customs. The books that record this knowledge, the *Vedas*, were probably first written around the time of this invasion; Ayurveda probably developed from the book known as the *Atharva Veda*.

Around 1000 B.C., knowledge in the classical texts of Ayurveda was further refined, giving rise to two textbooks, the *Charaka Samhita* and, much later, the *Sushruta Samhita*. This knowledge was further systematized in the Pauranic period (seventh century B.C.), when a text was produced on *Swastha-Vritta* or "Regimen for Health." This deals with *dinacharya* (daily routine) and *ritucharya* (seasonal adaptation). There is also a text known as the *Atur-Vritta* — "Regimen in Disease" — in which over 1000 diseases are described.

BUDDHISM AND AYURVEDA

Next came the Buddhist period, when knowledge of Ayurveda improved greatly. This was a golden age for this part of

Asia; even in the sixth century B.C. a "university," which became a center of medical science, existed at Taxila near Rawalpindi. There is a story about one of the students, Jivaka, who was dispatched by his teacher to go and find a plant that could not be used as a medicine. He was unable to do so, and was later appointed by King Bimbisara as his royal physician, responsible for the well-being of the Buddha and his disciples. The royal physician was very important for the stability of the state and thus highly respected. His endorsement by both the king and the Buddha ensured his success — people came from far and wide to be disciples of the Buddha just in order to be treated by the royal physician.

Although the Greeks were probably aware of Indian culture and their medical systems, the invasion of northern India by Alexander the Great in 326 B.C. was likely to have been responsible for the spread of Ayurveda into Europe. Once again, endorsement was the key factor; Alexander believed the system to be very effective. Meanwhile, in northern India, an emperor named Ashoka was also at work disseminating the ayurvedic system. He established a local network of hospitals and was very active in foreign relations, sending envoys with news of Ayurveda to bordering countries. A book on diagnostics appeared in the eighth century and the Buddhist movement set up universities to teach Buddhism, the wisdom recorded in the vedas, and other subjects, including medicine. One of these, Nalanda university, thrived until about the twelfth century.

THE END OF THE GOLDEN AGE

This golden age came to an end when northern India was invaded again. The invaders destroyed the universities and burned the libraries. Some Buddhist monks escaped to Tibet; a number of ayurvedic texts are preserved now only in a Tibetan translation. Nonetheless, Ayurveda survived as a system of medical practice, and documentation was maintained and added to as the centuries passed. In the medieval period (sometime between the twelfth and fifteenth centuries) a new textbook, the *Sarangakhara Samhita*, mentioned for the first time pulse examination and its relation to the diagnosis of diseases. Then, during the sixteenth century, Akbar the Mogul emperor organized the unification of all Indian medical systems.

Indian spices had been highly treasured in Europe for many centuries, and as trade routes opened up during the sixteenth and seventeenth centuries, Europeans developed a taste for anything Indian. During their colonial rule of India, the British used local ayurvedic medicines because of the expense and difficulty of importing Western medicine. However, the edict in 1835 that only European knowledge should be taught, together with the production of the British pharmacopoeia in 1858, caused many physicians to move away from the use of local drugs. Furthermore, the state no longer funded ayurvedic training and over the next century much knowledge and understanding were lost. Fortunately the textbooks survived, and European surgeons translated and brought into practice a technique described in the *Sushruta Samhita* to repair damage to the face. This technique fostered the discipline we now call plastic surgery.

AYURVEDA TODAY

Since Indian independence in 1947, Ayurveda has received recognition throughout India and is one of the six systems officially recognized by the country's government. Qualified ayurvedic physicians have been, and are being, registered as medical practitioners. A number of hospitals are already established in which patients are treated according to ayurvedic tenets, and practical lessons are given to students.

3

THE PHILOSOPHY
OF AYURVEDA

To understand Ayurveda it is important to understand something about its philosophy. Ayurveda is based on the Indian *samkhya* philosophy of creation. *Samkhya* comes from two Sanskrit words: *sat*, meaning "truth" and *khya*, meaning" to know."

A central theme of *samkhya* philosophy is that the one absolute truth is absolute consciousness, an idea very similar to modern views about the origin of our universe. Absolute consciousness represents a singularity. In the beginning, there was only one single essence. There was at that time no "existence" — there was no *thing* in the universe. Even the universe did not exist! The universe is considered to be an expression of that singularity. In samkhya philosophy there is a basic belief that the observable universe is only one of many manifestations of the absolute reality (in Sanskrit, *paramatma*). The *paramatma* is not limited in any way. Everything else in the universe, which is an expression of that reality, is limited. This is because the universe is constructed of opposites such as light and dark, near and far, and so on. In other words, we exist in a dualistic universe rather than in a singularity. Words are dualistic and limited, and we use words to describe everything. However, because everything is a representation of the absolute, the truth exists already within all things, including human beings; it simply has to be realized and brought forth. This truth includes the information required for healing. We only have to discover and realize it.

AYURVEDIC PHILOSOPHY

According to *samkhya* philosophy, the primary force that pervades the universe is consciousness; matter arises from consciousness, not vice versa. All of creation is present only to glorify the absolute reality or absolute self. It is our illusion that the universe is stable; as we all now know, it appears to be constantly expanding and, if there is enough matter in the universe it will eventually slow down and collapse again to a singularity.

Samkhya philosophy also states that the universe will go on collapsing and re-expanding over and over again forever. The universe is governed by a set of rules, of which the most important perhaps is that all "things" come to pass. Put another way, everything is constantly changing regardless of the illusion of stability. It is only God, or the absolute reality, which is beyond change.

People are not excluded from this rule of change; our bodies are constantly changing (albeit apparently slowly), as are our minds and our beliefs, with every new experience or piece of information that comes our way. Our environment is also changing, but it is made up of the same chemical elements as our physical form; the energy within the universe is no different than that in our minds. The aim of Ayurveda is to make sure that there is internal harmony and that the internal is in complete harmony with the environment at every level.

It is said in *samkha* philosophy that until the "singularity," or absolute consciousness, desires to experience itself, it remains a singularity. In addition, because desire is the causative agent that brought the universe into being, it pervades all things. It generates duality from unity. The Genesis story in the Bible tells essentially the same story: God divided the heavens from the earth and the light from the dark, and so on, implying that originally they were one.

PRAKRUTI

The primary aspect of the created universe is nature, or *prakruti* in Sanskrit; it is the complicated web of the manifested universe. It is this difference between absolute reality and nature that gives rise to the feeling of separateness—that "I" am different from the person next door or playing a different role than "I" was yesterday. This "I" is known as the "go," or in Sanskrit the *ahamkara*. The *ahamkara* "I" represents the physical and chemical components and processes of the body, as opposed to the true "I," the soul, or that part of a being that is an unchangeable part of the truth of creation, known in Sanskrit as the *Atman*.

THE GUNAS

Ahamkara, or the biochemical and physical processes of the body, may be considered as composed of an in-built, all encompassing order or equilibrium. The energy that creates this equilibrium has three qualities known as *gunas*. They are: *sattva* (sometimes translated as purity and also as subjective consciousness); *rajas* (activity, passion, the process of change); and *tamas* (darkness, inertia). In the human being, *sattva* is the ability of the five senses to react in the way they do; it is not the sense organs themselves or the process of nervous impulses traveling to the brain, but simply the *abil-*

ity of those sense organs to be able to sense what is available to be sensed. *Tamas* represents all that has form and inertia, or resistance to being moved. In the case of the sense organs, *tamas* represents their physical structure. *Rajas* is the kinetic energy that links together *tamas* and *sattva*; for example, it includes the movement of impulses from the sense organs to the brain.

According to *samkhya*, these three *gunas* are continually separating and uniting, and are present in varying proportions in everything that makes up the physical world. Together they create the first cosmic soundless sound, AUM (OM), which continually operates in this universe.

We shall look at each of the *gunas* in turn and explore how they contribute to the world we perceive.

SATTVA

The expression of the soul that is part of, and continuous with, absolute consciousness is determined by the state of health of the body; the soul itself remains pure and unaffected. It is only its expression in the outside world that is modified by health or illness. *Sattva* is the essence of what is needed to make you and me the way we are, or at least the way we are meant to be — pure consciousness and bliss.

RAJAS

Rajas represents action or movement. It is an expression of all transfers of energy from one state to another, of all living metabolic processes and of all our physical activities. It provides the link between *tamas* (matter or inertia) and *sattva* (the subjective consciousness); it connects subject with object. *Rajas* and *sattva* unite together to produce eleven sense and motor organs that are the functioning structure of the human body.

While *sattva* and *tamas* are fundamental, *rajas* is a linking power; there would be no "experience" if the force of *rajas* was not present to enable the expression of the other two. It is the quality of this vital coexistent balance that is the central tenet of Ayurveda.

TAMAS

Tamas is divided into five principle parts that give form to the five senses: sound, touch, form, taste and odor. These in turn give form to the division of the elements that make up the universe.

They are:

- ether
- air
- fire
- water
- earth

These are the elements of the environment and of ourselves.

THE FIVE ELEMENTS

Earth has the character of *solidity.*

Water has the character of *liquidity.*

Air has the character of *gas.*

Fire has the character of *change / energy.*

Ether has the character of *space.*

Ether is a difficult concept for us in the West to grasp. It is hard to understand how the space in which other things exist can have a physical form — there appears to be nothing in it by definition. Yet space is a part of physical creation. Remember that we used to believe the Sun rotated around the Earth, but now appreciate that the reverse is true. If the universe is expanding, what is it expanding into, if not space? The answer is that more space is created as the universe expands — it does not exist outside the universe.

Imagine that you are at the North Pole painting concentric circles on the ice, standing on unpainted ice outside your circles. Paint more circles and eventually you will arrive at the South Pole; you are now standing at the South Pole on the inside of your circles! Extend this concept to a golf ball and cover it with coats of paint. If you keep on doing this it will eventually reach almost the size of the universe. At this point, by analogy with the paint circles on the earth, you will find yourself painting on the inside.

In other words, space is a physical feature of the universe and does not exist outside it — it is finite. Modern physics theory predicts, but has not yet proven, that all matter is composed of identical elementary particles. If shown to be true, then the same theory predicts that space will also be composed of the same particles. Therefore space, at the finest level of discrimination, has a physical form. This physical concept of space is synonymous with what is known in Ayurveda as "ether."

In Ayurveda, a person is composed of these five elements plus consciousness. Given that it is our nature to be pure consciousness and bliss, and that the expression of the soul or consciousness is affected by the state of health of our bodies, you would expect that devotion to well-being should be our primary objective. Unfortunately, it is so often the third or fourth objective in our daily lives.

Desire is said to have caused the universe to spring into existence, probably because of an imbalance in the original singularity. Desire is also the force that causes imbalance in the body and thus "illness"; this is especially true of selfish desire (in Sanskrit, *raga*). One of the desires of modern man is to live as long as possible, but this ignores the possibility of living well. Ayurveda is concerned with living well, not necessarily with living longer; if the latter is the result of living well, that is fine, but it should not be a primary desire in itself. Given the choice of another forty years of life wracked with pain or twenty years of pure bliss, which would you choose?

Living well implies achieving balance within the body, mind and spirit, preventing disease from arising rather than attempting to cure it once it has arisen. It is a way of life involving balance in diet, work, play and rest. Only by applying the appropriate measure of each of these ingredients will internal and external harmony be achieved. Ayurveda enables us to be aware of what we need and of what we do not need, and thus make informed choices for ourselves as to how to live and remain healthy.

4

HOW DOES
AYURVEDA WORK?

In Ayurveda, health is defined as perfect balance between body, mind, spirit and the environment; ayurvedic techniques focus on achieving that balance. Balance is achieved by the correct "measure" of all things, although there is a thin line between enough and too much. Our desires usually cause us to lose sight of the correct measure in a particular circumstance; the most common desires causing this problem are those such as lust, hatred, fear, envy, arrogance or greed. The loss of measure causes imbalance in our lives.

We do most things in our lives because of one desire or another, and not just desires such as lust; there are four other fundamental desires:

- to live to see another day, and ultimately as many days as possible

- to do what we were born to do (whatever we may believe that to be) — *dharma* in Sanskrit

- to have enough resources, usually money (*artha* in Sanskrit), to perform our *dharma* or destiny

- to be happy (we imagine by achievement of the previous three) — *sukha* in Sanskrit

This set of needs has been redefined in modern times by Abraham Maslow and presented as a "hierarchy of needs."

Desire causes lack of measure, which results in imbalance of the body and mind and so leads to disease; if everything is in balance then health prevails. We all know happy people who appear to be well most of the time and, conversely, sad people who seem to be ill all of the time. An important path toward happiness and good health is liberation from the mind, where all our desires arise. But sadly, the mind and its desires control our actions, rule our lives and cause imbalance.

However, we all as children learned the truism "too much of a good thing is bad for you" and most of us know (usually after too much rich food) how accurate this is. How do we balance the way we lead our lives by always applying measure to everything we do and how can we discover what that measure is?

THE DOSHAS

In control of the living processes of the mind and body, and responsible for achieving and maintaining balance are three principle "energies," or doshas. The Sanskrit word *dosha* is the root of the Greek prefix *dys*, used in English words such as dysentery or dysfunction, meaning "fault." These three doshas are called *pitta*, *vata* and *kapha* and they are arranged as follows:

- *pitta* — a combination of fire and water

- *vata* — a combination of air and ether

- *kapha* — a combination of water and earth

The state of perfect health is bliss or total "stillness," but the nature of life is one of action and movement. So how can this bliss be achieved when our bodies and minds are vitalized by these three "out of balance" forces? It is perhaps easiest to consider the state of body and mind as a triangle, with *vata*, *pitta* and *kapha* pulling or pushing at each of the three corners respectively. If the three forces are in balance the triangle will remain perfectly still, whereas if one or more of them are out of balance with the others then the triangle will move in the direction of the forces pulling the strongest. In both the body and the mind, this loss of stability, or disharmony, causes disease. The doshas each have specific activities in the body. *Vata* is responsible for motion in both the body and the mind. *Pitta* is in charge of any form of change. *Kapha* produces lubrication as well as insulation.

GENERAL FUNCTIONS OF THE THREE DOSHAS

All bodies are made up of combinations of these elements and their resultant forces, as is our food or anything else we come into contact with.

When we are in balance the five elements function together healthily; when they are out of balance and the "triangle" is biased in one direction or another the body appears to function abnormally and we become ill. It is important to understand that the doshas, while essential for the vital force of life, are themselves "faults." There is more than one level of balance. It is not sufficient, in the event of imbalance due to an excess of one *dosha*, to increase the other two believing that equilibrium will be restored. What is necessary is to decrease the influence of the one that is in excess.

Kapha

Kapha is largely occupied in the manufacture of slippery, oily, thick, tenacious substances. These lubricating, protective and adhesive compounds are essential to untroubled daily life; they ease the movements of one surface over another without friction and prevent entry of harmful bacteria and dust to the body. If *kapha* is inadequately cleared from the body or if there is an excess intake, an excess of these materials, such as mucus, develops. If this excess is not cleared it leads to disease or increased susceptibility to disease, such as sinusitis. Insufficient *kapha* intake will result in dryness, not due to an excess of air but rather to inadequate lubrication, resulting in roughness, discomfort and instability. Some forms of arthritis are the result of *kapha* disorders.

GENERAL FUNCTIONS OF THE THREE DOSHAS		
Vata	*Pitta*	*Kapha*
• transmission of nerve impulses	• digestion of food	• mucus in the gut to lubricate food movement
• circulation of blood through the heart and body	• metabolism	• mucus in the airways to ease respiration and trap dust particles
• breathing	• production of body heat	
• transport of secretions from all the glands	• discrimination	• synovial fluid to lubricate the joints
• movement of food through the gut	• vision	• physical matter in the body
• excretion of urine and feces	• color of the skin and eyes	• insulation
• childbirth	• production of hunger and thirst	• staying power
• expression of emotion	• conversion of sensation into nerve impulses	• sleep
• vitality	• thought processes	• long-term memory
• creativity	• appreciation	• flexibility of tissues
• enthusiasm	• reasoning	• compassion
	• intelligence	• patience and stability
	• confidence	

Pitta

Pitta is concerned with digestion and is responsible for the production of stomach acid and biliary secretions vital to the breakdown of food. Bile is, however, always excreted ultimately along with the remainder of digestive waste products via the feces. In the event of obstruction or slower-than-normal excretion of the feces, the bile is reabsorbed and creates a "hot" condition, or inflammation in the body. Excessive production of *pitta* creates excess acid and bile, associated with burning sensations in the gut and in the mind, with a bilious nature. Inadequate intake/production of *pitta* results in so-called "cold" diseases — a lack of energy and confidence.

Vata

One of the end products of *vata* is gas in the body, but it is more significantly the motive force behind all transmission of nervous impulses both in the brain and the peripheral nerves. Excessive nervous activity is seen as over-sensitivity and we often refer in a derogatory manner to people with excess *vata* in the brain as "air-heads" or "spaced out." The expression of emotions may be inappropriate and the heart rate unsuited to the needs of the circulation. We would term someone with too much *vata* as "being of a nervous disposition." It cannot be a comfortable way to exist.

The doshas are not in themselves entities such as enzymes, air or mucus. They are simply forces pulling on the corners of the triangle. They are rather like high and low pressure zones in the atmosphere; apart from the weather forecasters' map, we cannot see the different pressures, but we do feel the winds that they cause and see things moving in the breeze. The doshas have principle locations in the body: *kapha* is located mainly above the diaphragm; *vata* below the navel, especially in the colon and bladder; and *pitta* lies in between these two in the region of the liver. Each of the three forces also predominate in specific organs, sometimes just one and sometimes two are in the majority. Although it is only in the body and mind overall that balance exists, each individual tissue expresses a variation in representation of the doshas which is suited to the nature of that tissue and represents "balance" for that organ.

PREDOMINANCE OF THE DOSHAS		
Vata	*Pitta*	*Kapha*
nerves	brain	brain
brain	liver	joints
spinal cord	spleen	mouth
heart	small intestine	head
ears	endocrine glands	neck
skin	skin	stomach
lungs	eyes	lymph
bones	blood	lungs
	sweat	heart
		esophagus
		fat

FUNCTIONS OF THE DOSHAS

The three doshas are further divided into five categories each, by reference to their specific functions. (See "Function of the Doshas" on the next page).

Vata, being the power behind all things moving, is classified in a slightly different way. First, *prana vata*, being a forward moving force, is situated between the diaphragm and the throat; *udana vata* is positioned between the throat and head and termed upward moving; *samana vata*, an "equalizing" air, exists between the diaphragm and the navel; *apana vata* is downward moving and in the lower abdomen; lastly, *vyana vata* pervades everything and is distributed throughout the core of the body.

FUNCTIONS OF THE DOSHAS	
Kapha	*Pitta*
stomach mucus (*kledak*)	digestive juices (*pachaka*)
pleural and pericardial fluid (*avalambak*)	hemoglobin (*ranjak*)
	melanin (*bhrajak*)
saliva (*bodhak*)	rhodopsin (*alochak*)
synovial fluid (*sleshak*)	neurotransmitters (*sadhak*)
cerebrospinal fluid (*tarpak*)	

THE LIVING PROCESS AND THE ENVIRONMENT

Everything entering the body — heat, light, sound, thoughts, experiences and food — must be first digested by the application of "fire" (*agni* in Sanskrit) otherwise it will end up in a form that is unsuitable and will cause disease. For example, digestion normally breaks down all proteins into small fragments that can safely be absorbed. The poisonous nature of some deadly mushrooms is due to the fact that some of their proteins are very unusual and the digestive process is unable to break them down properly. As a result, they are absorbed undigested, and the presence of these foreign proteins in the body causes a severe reaction. If properly broken down, they would be nutritious rather than deadly. If everything is correctly "digested," the doshas remain in balance. But if there is inadequate digestion (a weak or faulty *agni*), then an imbalance in the doshas is caused and disease will follow. This is another part of the vicious circle, for an imbalance in the doshas tends to cause weak or faulty *agni*. The effects of individual doshas on the nature of this digestive fire, which applies as much to the music we listen to as the food we eat, is as follows:

- increased *vata* makes the digestive fire behave erratically, just like a wind blowing on a bonfire — one is never sure which way it will blow next and it can become unpredictable and dangerous

- increased *pitta* makes the fire fiercer, just like throwing gasoline on a bonfire — the fire becomes much hotter, larger and all consuming

- increased *kapha* dulls the fire — just like throwing water or dirt on a bonfire; the flames die down and it looks as though the fire may go out at any moment; it may also take a long time to recover.

WASTE DISPOSAL MECHANISM

The doshas also affect every other process in the body, and for the ayurvedic physician the next most important system is the primary waste disposal mechanism — the lower bowel and the production of feces. All the processes in the large bowel, including excretion, are very important to our health.

Disturbances of this function inevitably give rise to problems elsewhere. Increased *vata* here causes, as one might expect, erratic bowel movements ranging from constipation to diarrhea. Increased *pitta* causes bowel motions to be soft and loose, but without the frequency or explosive nature of diarrhea. *Kapha* excess has very little adverse effect here.

THE INDIVIDUAL CONSTITUTION

Every person is created different from the next — we all have our individual constitutions. Our unique characteristics are said to be generated at the moment of conception and relate to the constitutions of each parent, their thoughts and emotional attitude (*bhawana* in Sanskrit), the time of year and the environment. This basic fixed constitution with which we are born is called the *prakruti*. The dependence upon conditions at the time of conception is why parents are advised to avoid noxious substances such as alcohol and tobacco prior to the time of conception; this caution should also be extended to the state of mind and the environment at the time. This basic constitution expresses itself in the nature of people as follows.

INDIVIDUAL CONSTITUTION			
Dosha:	Vata	Pitta	Kapha
Nature	erratic	intense	laid back
Result	unable to retain mass and dissipates energy	tendency to excess control of both energy and mass	retains mass easily with poor expression of energy

There are eight possible combinations of these doshas, making up the basic constitutional types:

Vata

Pitta

Kapha

Vata + Pitta

Pitta + Kapha

Kapha + Vata

Vata + Pitta + Kapha (unbalanced)

Vata + Pitta + Kapha (balanced)

The ideal constitution is when all three doshas are present and in balance; sadly, this is very unusual.

Conversely, the unbalanced vata+ pitta+ kapha constitution is almost always associated with constant health problems. The majority of us have a prakruti predominated by two doshas and a few have single dosha constitutions. Those with a dual prakruti, while not as prone to ill health as the out-of-balance tridoshic individuals, are nonetheless much more difficult to treat than those with a single doshic make-up.

For them, disease may arise not only from each *dosha*, individually, but also from the combination of the two.

THE CURRENT (DAY-TO-DAY) CONSTITUTION (VIKRUTI)

The maintenance of balance is the primary goal of Ayurveda. The secondary goal is to bring back into balance what has gone "out of whack" so that it may then be *kept* in balance. The current ratio of the doshas in the individual from day to day, known as the *vikruti*, is created by the food eaten, literature read, conversation, music, thoughts and so on. To achieve internal balance it is best if the *vikruti* is identical to the *prakruti*. The ayurvedic principle in this respect is that like increases like; thus a diet high in *pitta* will tend to increase the *pitta* imbalance in someone who has a *pitta prakruti* and conversely a diet low in *pitta* will tend to reduce the *pitta* factor in that person.

If we dive into a cold swimming pool or into the sea the water temperature eventually makes us feel cold and will ultimately drop our body temperature. When we come out we shiver, creating a marked rise in metabolic activity (*pitta*), increasing again the heat within ourselves. Alternatively, we may go into a sauna and heat flows into our bodies, raising the temperature toward normal. Perhaps more importantly, in the sauna we "feel" hot in the same way that we "feel" cold under a cold shower. The child with a raging temperature is sponged with tepid water to bring the temperature down to a safe level. Thought also affects the functioning of the body; anger, anxiety and frustration are often associated with stomach ulcers and the pain from them, and vice versa. Pain does not have the effect of making us feel happy; we feel emotions and process our thoughts very differently depending upon whether we feel hot, cold or comfortable. In short, everything has its effect upon everything else and because of this we can take steps to alter our *vikruti* if we wish.

We are what we think we are. We are what we eat. We are what we do. So we have it within our power to choose to be healthy and ultimately to experience peace and bliss. To do this, we need to explore in some detail the nature of the items we eat and our everyday experiences so that we can predict whether they will each tend to worsen or improve the imbalance we have; it is quite rare to find an individual whose *vikruti* is similar to their *prakruti*. We all have to work at it consciously.

QUALITIES OF MATTER

In Ayurveda, there are ten basic pairs of qualities that describe the nature of all things — actions, substances, time and space:

1. Heavy / light
2. Dull / intense
3. Hot / cold
4. Oily / dry
5. Smooth / rough
6. Soft / hard
7. Stable / mobile
8. Subtle / gross
9. Solid / liquid
10. Clear / sticky

The most significant of these qualities are hot/cold, heavy/light and oily/dry.

Both the quality of a food and the strength of our digestion determine the effect of any of these upon our *dosha* balance. Their effect is also related to our current state, or *vikruti*. Coming into a warm house from cold weather outside gives us the impression that the house is hot, whereas coming into a warm house when it is hot outside elicits the response that the house feels pleasantly cool. In the same way, people with different constitutions (*prakruti*) respond very differently when placed in the same environment. This is why some of us "feel the cold" more than others.

DIGESTION

Food, or any other "input" for that matter, has to be digested by the body. The results of food digestion are substances known in Sanskrit as *dhatus*, which are used to build the tissues of the body.

In Ayurveda, there is a sequence to the production of various elements that compose the body, with sundry waste products being produced along the way. The nutritional essence from the digested food is used to produce the first *dhatu*; the nutritional essence from this *dhatu* is transformed to produce the next *dhatu* in the sequence and so on. This is seen as a continual process of refinement, in that the "essence" is refined each time. At each step of refinement, waste products are produced and expelled in one form or another from the body.

Nutrition begins when the first elements of "essence" are extracted from the food by the digestive processes in the intestines. These elements become something referred to as *rasa*, meaning "anything nourishing." This extraction into *rasa* is slightly different from what we in the West understand by digestion; it applies not only to the physical/chemical components of the food but also to its appearance, taste, texture, color and odor. The same is true for all experience: everything we have an interaction with has these qualities, even though they may not have a biochemical structure that can be eaten. The color of the room in which you are sitting or the clothes you are wearing at this moment, the sounds you can hear, the fragrances in the air, the words you are reading, the movement of air and the sensations of touch are all affecting your mind and body and are being converted into the *dhatus* of the body at every moment.

Modern intensive care units in hospitals play music to patients in a coma because they appear to recover more rapidly than if they are surrounded by silence. The latest research has shown that playing Baroque music at a low volume increases the ability of the mind to learn and retain what it is reading during the time the music is playing. It seems that the patterns in Baroque music are very similar to activity in those parts of the brain responsible for retention and recall; the external patterns are "nourishing" and reinforce the patterns in the brain. In other words, similar qualities have a reinforcing effect on one another. This is in accordance with Ayurveda's principle tenet that like increases like and conversely that dislike causes reduction.

We have control over everything in our realm of experience if we choose to have control. And, the easiest to control and perhaps the most significant influence on our experience of the external environment is food. If you live in a climate that is not suited to your constitution (or *prakruti*), there may be little that can be done to change it apart from moving, an option not open to most people. However, we *can* adjust what we eat to offset the adverse effect of the climate or environmental factors that cannot be controlled.

THE QUALITIES OF FOOD

Food has three main qualities — its taste, its strength and its effect. Of these, taste is extremely important because it has a marked effect upon the *rasa* produced. So eating different tastes will affect the personality and the health of the body regardless of the number of calories or amount of protein present. The body needs and indeed may actually crave certain tastes in order to achieve contentment and good health. There is a catch here, however, for there is a tendency for us to be unable to separate the cravings of the body from those of the mind! The mind can be our friend but also our enemy. The mind can be the greatest craver of all and it usually craves all the wrong things. The distinction between these two cravings is perhaps the most crucial step that we need to take in order to modify our health and well-being.

The tastes associated with food are: sweet, sour, salty, bitter, pungent and astringent. Pungent means sharp, burning or strong in food terms (caustic when referring to speech). Astringent is derived from the Latin *ad* plus *stringere*, meaning "to draw tight"; it is akin to the sensation experienced when eating unripe bananas or pomegranates — they cause the mouth to pucker (in speech, the descriptive terms "stern" or "austere" are probably more appropriate).

These tastes have different effects upon the doshas as follows:

- decreasing *vata*: sweet, sour, salty
- decreasing *pitta*: sweet, bitter, astringent (if *pitta* increased)
- decreasing *kapha*: pungent, bitter, astringent (if *kapha* increased)
- increasing *vata*: pungent, astringent, bitter (in excess)
- increasing *pitta*: sour, salty, pungent
- increasing *kapha*: sweet, sour, salty

The strength of something is related to its "taste," but not necessarily to the sensation perceived upon the tongue. "Sweet" foods are more strengthening than sour foods, in the same way as beautiful art, music or words are "stronger" than discordant music or art. The hierarchical order of strengths of the various tastes are sweet, sour, salty, bitter, pungent and, weakest of all, astringent.

By taking into account all the properties of the foods we eat and the activities we perform, it is possible to adjust them so that there will be an effect upon the *vikruti*, or our current constitution.

Lack of attention to these matters frequently leads to imbalance in the doshas, and as a result the digestive and metabolic fire (*agni*) in various parts of the body becomes disturbed. If this fire of life is disturbed, it will not function correctly; the result is the production of improperly digested food or incorrect metabolism, culminating in the creation of *ama*. *Ama* is undigested food or a substance produced by inappropriate metabolism at any level — it is the cause of all disease. Imbalance in the mind due to emotional attachments also causes *ama*, which gives rise to mental disease. Mental imbalances can become physical ones and vice versa.

The term "imbalance" in the doshas means a difference of your current constitution and that which is your basic nature, or *prakruti*. This imbalance affects digestion and metabolism, but is of relatively little consequence until the *ama* produced begins to "settle in" or affect a tissue of the body, usually one that already has a predisposing weakness. For a while, the tissue is relatively unaffected, but as time goes by the presence of increasing amounts of *ama* in the tissue leads to gross symptoms of disease. If these are allowed to go unheeded, then ultimately the *ama* "overflows" from this tissue and you begin to experience symptoms in other tissues of the body or in the mind.

Ama is considered to be the principle cause of disease, though illness can arise in other ways as well. For example, a considerable excess of *kapha* in the body can act to block the movement of *vata*. Movement of one sort or another is, as we all know, vital for the processes in the body and when it is "blocked" it often gives rise to pain.

The theory behind the cause of disease in the ayurvedic system is simple and straightforward. However, in practice it can be extremely complex. For this reason, it is advisable to consult an ayurvedic physician to obtain an accurate and early diagnosis. The physician will be able to detect imbalances in the doshas and rebalance them, thus preventing future disease. The physician will also be able to distinguish disease and the symptoms caused by accumulation of *ama* from those caused by severe doshic imbalance. There are, however, many things you can do yourself to balance the doshas and prevent, or even cure, disease.

5

A PERSONAL STEP-BY-STEP GUIDE

In order to decide upon the most appropriate lifestyle for yourself, the first thing to do is to determine, as accurately as possible, your *prakruti*, or basic constitution. There are many ways to accomplish this and it is probably best to use all of them rather than opt for one or two things that may miss the whole picture. Read the descriptions below and answer the questions that follow each section honestly. Do not be tempted to choose a characteristic because it appears to "fit in" with others or because you see one as "preferable" to another. This can be very difficult! It may be best to ask a friend to complete the questions for you. If there is a question that you cannot answer leave it blank.

BODY FRAME

People with a *vata* constitution are often very tall or very short. They are usually thin and somewhat gawky, have a small body frame with narrow shoulders and hips and have delicate wrists and ankles. They are rather delicate, with limbs that seem too thin for their length and they frequently benefit from thin, tapering fingers. There may be disproportion in the body make-up, such that some parts seem light and others heavy. It is the nature of *vata* to be unpredictable. Owing to a lack of fatty tissues, particularly just under the skin, the wrists, knees, ankles and elbows may seem to stick out or be knobby. Joints such as knees or elbows often "click" when straightened. Any unusual bony features are usually indicative of the influence of *vata*. The absence of subcutaneous fat means that veins and tendons are also plainly visible. If you have many of these characteristics there is a strong *vata* element in you.

If you have a medium frame with average shoulders and hips, there is a strong *pitta* element in your constitution. Fingers and toes are neither skinny nor pudgy and are of average length. Everything is in proportion and naturally slightly athletic.

Kapha-predominant people have a medium-to-large frame with large bones, broad shoulders and wide hips. *Kapha* qualities are water and earth, stability and reserve, so it is not surprising that these people tend to be large and bulky. Football players are classically composed of this type of individual. The body proportions are in balance and all on the large side, the bones do not stick out, nor are the joints visible. The fingers and toes are often quite short and plump, the neck robust.

Please mark the features that best describe you. Key features are marked with a ".

BODY FRAME			
Characteristic:	Vata	Pitta	Kapha
Size at birth«	❏ Small	❏ Medium	❏ Large
Height«	❏ Exceptionally short or tall	❏ Average	❏ Short and stocky; tall and large
Anatomical features«	❏ Bony joints that crack, prominent veins	❏ Well proportioned	❏ Broad shoulders, strong muscles

WEIGHT

Vata types are usually thin. These are the people who eat vast amounts of food, go back for seconds and have dessert, yet never seem to put on one ounce in weight! Everyone else envies them but seldom understands that the *vata* person is actually trying to put on a little weight and is extremely frustrated because he or she cannot, however much he or she tries. All of the energy from the food is spent in nervous energy and movement both inside and outside the body so there is nothing left to store as fat. *Vata* types are often referred to as "skin and bones." One of the reasons they stay this way is because their diet is often fairly balanced regardless of quantity. However, the desire to gain weight can lead to eating a diet designed solely for weight gain and is therefore unbalanced. In this way, it is possible for some *vata* types to become overweight and almost certainly ill at the same time. If a good diet is resumed, they can quite easily lose the excess weight and recover an overall sense of well-being.

Pitta people find it easy to keep their weight steady and are usually in the middle of the ideal weight for height tables. They do not develop midriff bulges if they put on weight but tend to distribute the weight evenly over the body. *Pitta* is the fire/metabolism/balance force in the constitution and so they can put on weight if they wish to, or lose it by increasing exercise if required.

On the other hand, those with a *kapha* constitution need to exercise if they are to keep their weight at a reasonable level. They are generally heavier for a given height than the other two classes. These are the people who can gain weight just by looking at a piece of cake. They find it difficult to lose the weight they have put on over the years, very often on the buttocks and legs. It is their nature to store energy as fat and be heavy. Ultimately, if the process is allowed to continue the deposition of fat will begin to involve the other areas of the body as well. When the time comes to lose weight they find that it disappears from the top half of the torso, then the waist, but seems to be almost impossible to lose around the buttocks and legs.

Please mark the feature that *best* describes you.

WEIGHT			
Characteristic:	*Vata*	*Pitta*	*Kapha*
Weight	❏ Light, hard to gain weight	❏ Moderate, gains and loses weight easily	❏ Heavy, difficulty losing weight

HAIR

To some extent, as with skin color, the nature of your head hair is related to your racial background. So it is important to assess your hair as similar, straighter or curlier than one might anticipate given the average nature of hair in your racial group.

Vata people have dry hair on their heads more often than not. However, as with the skin, it may be variable across the scalp. It is seldom naturally blond and tends to have a coarse or rough texture. It is usually quite curly and occasionally frizzy or tightly kinked. Dandruff is common. Because the hair also lacks emollients to keep it supple and shiny, the *vata* individual suffers split ends and dry, lackluster hair. Body hair is either sparse or in excess — dark, rough and curly.

Pitta is the fire principle and fire is red, so if you have naturally red hair *pitta* features strongly in your *prakruti*. If *pitta* people are not red-headed, they have blond or light brown hair, or hair that turns gray or white as early as their twenties. Premature hair loss in men is also a feature of strong *pitta*. The hair is usually thin and fine, quite straight and almost impossible to style without the use of hair gel or body enhancers. The high output of oils by the *pitta* skin on the scalp can result in the hair being so oily that it appears flat; in addition, dust may stick readily to this excess oil and cause dullness. Body hair is also white to light brown in color and very fine.

Hair that is brown to dark brown, thick and slightly wavy rather than really curly (see *vata* hair above) is characteristic of the *kapha* influence. There is usually a moderate amount of body hair.

Please mark the features that *best* describe you.

HAIR			
Characteristic:	*Vata*	*Pitta*	*Kapha*
Hair color (relative)"	❏ Very dark	❏ Fair/red/ light brown	❏ Medium brown
Hair thickness"	❏ Medium	❏ Fine	❏ Thick
Texture"	❏ Coarse	❏ Silky	❏ Soft
Form"	❏ Curly	❏ Straight	❏ Wavy

NAILS

Hard, brittle nails that crack and split easily with ridges are suggestive of a *vata prakruti*. As always, irregularity of size and structure is typical of vata. Nail biters and pencil chewers are usually *vata* types. The nails of a *pitta* person are soft, but strong and smooth. The nail bed tends to be reddish in color. *Kapha* nails are strong, large, thick and regular. The thickness may cause the nail bed to appear pale.

Please mark the features that *best* describe you.

Nails			
Characteristic:	*Vata*	*Pitta*	*Kapha*
Nail color	❏ Pale	❏ Red	❏ Opaque
Nail strength	❏ Brittle	❏ Strong	❏ Tough
Nail size	❏ Irregular and ridged	❏ Regular	❏ Regular/ almost square

Eyes

Eye color is not easily determined for some people; in answering the following questions use the underlying eye color and ignore any small spots or flecks. Also, remember that once again different races tend to have specific ranges of eye color and your answers must be in relation to that range. Eye size is subjective, so you may wish to ask someone else to comment on the size of your eyes as well as how much they normally move.

Vata constitutional eyes are characteristically gray to gray-blue in the iris (the circle around the black pupil) but can also be very dark brown; if you have eyes of different colors then the variable influence of *vata* is at work again. *Vata* people's eyes are often "dry" and frequently feel as though there is something caught under the eyelid. They can seem somewhat dull and are usually a little small. They appear constantly on the move, darting from one side to the other, apparently tirelessly, but are in fact consuming energy under the influence of *vata*, which is thus not available to be converted into fat.

The eyes of the *pitta* person generally range from hazel through green to light blue, including iridescent blue. They are medium in size and easily inflamed. Indeed, even during good health there are usually one or two blood vessels visible in the sclera (the white part around the iris). *Pitta* eyes have a sharp steady gaze and can be quite penetrating, seeming at times almost to have the power to burn a hole in the object or person being observed.

Large, moist, mid-brown/dark blue, olive shaped eyes are typical of the *kapha* constitution. Movement is neither rapid nor the gaze intense; these eyes seem to exude softness.

Please mark the features that *best* describe you.

EYES			
Characteristic:	Vata	Pitta	Kapha
Eye color (relative	❏ Dark brown or different	❏ Hazel, green, light blue, intense	❏ Mid brown/ dark blue
Eye size*	❏ Small	❏ Medium	❏ Large
Eye movement*	❏ Rapid and incessant	❏ Sharp, steady	❏ Slow

You may wish to ask someone else's opinion on these.

SKIN

Your skin color is determined largely by your parents' racial backgrounds and also by the nature of and your exposure to the environment in which you live. A northern European who seems well-tanned will still be very much lighter in skin tone than the palest person with an African heritage. This is a relative subject, and you need to compare your color to the members of your family and with others of your ethnicity in order to be accurate. It may be easier to ask one of your parents or friends from your racial group. It is not easy if your parents are from widely different racial backgrounds. If this is the case, it may be better not to answer the question on color.

Vata people are rather on the dark side compared to their compatriots; they tan easily and do not tend to burn. They love the sun and heat and are always seeking it; they get a buzz from being out in the sunlight. This is because *vata* is, by its very nature, cold; *vata*-dominated people do not store much energy to keep warm, so they actually need the heat. Their skin appears cold to other people, and often has a grayish hue. They always, with reason, complain that their circulation is bad and they suffer interminably from cold feet.

Pitta people generally have light-colored skin, often pinkish. They have a ruddy glow and are often covered in freckles; tanning is difficult for them — they burn readily and can suffer from unpleasant allergic reactions to sunlight. They have naturally warm/hot skin as perceived by others.

With *kapha* as your constitutional type you enjoy sunbathing, but can burn (though not as readily as *pitta* types). Your skin is cool—though not as cold as the *vata* person's to the touch—but cold hands and feet are unusual.

Please mark the features that *best* describe you.

SKIN			
Characteristic:	*Vata*	*Pitta*	*Kapha*
Skin color (relative)"	❏ Dark	❏ Fair	❏ "White"
Skin temperature*	❏ Cool	❏ Hot	❏ Warm
Tendency to burn"	❏ Low	❏ High	❏ Moderate
Tanning ability	❏ Easy	❏ Poor	❏ Moderately easy

Ask someone else to answer this one for you.

SKIN CHARACTERISTICS

Dry skin is the lot of the *vata* person. The constant movement and high energy expenditure means that the little moisture there is in the skin rapidly disappears. Once again, the unpredictable nature of *vata* comes into play and while some parts of the skin may be dry, others may be normal; if *vata* is particularly strong, the skin may be dry everywhere. A lack of lubricating, emollient substances in the skin results in cracking, peeling and, when exposed to the sun, a somewhat leathery or wrinkled appearance (though not burned). Cold weather can, paradoxically, have a similar effect on the *vata* skin—if you always have to apply additional lubricants to your lips in the winter to prevent them from drying out, then *vata* is in your primary constitution.

Pitta people frequently have fine skin, are somewhat prone to developing rashes and show a particular tendency to acne in adolescence and throughout their lives. Moles are common and, owing to the potentially increased rate of internal metabolism, the skin's elastic tissues develop problems earlier than most people's, meaning wrinkles appear sooner. *Pitta* people become flushed easily upon exertion — they actually look hot. As you might expect, blushing comes almost second nature to the *pitta*.

Individuals with a *kapha* constitution have somewhat oily, almost waxy, smooth, thick skin with few wrinkles. The skin is well supplied with emollients from the body's own sources. It is almost too uniform in terms of texture; this is not just because there is more subcutaneous fat underneath it, but rather *kapha*'s stable nature — the antithesis of *vata*.

Please mark the features that *best* describe you.

SKIN CHARACTERISTICS			
Characteristic:	Vata	Pitta	Kapha
Skin surface	❑ Dry, prone to chapping and psoriasis	❑ Fine, prone to acne and rashes	❑ Smooth and waxy
Wrinkles	❑ Fine, in sunlight	❑ Early	❑ Very few

SWEAT

Remember that this set of qualities and questions is aimed at your *prakruti*, or basic constitution, and not necessarily exactly how you are now; so it can be helpful to think back to when you were a child. If you have a marked imbalance now, resulting in an increase in weight and subcutaneous fat, then it may be that you have a tendency to sweat more than you used to. Try to answer this question by considering how you were in your childhood.

The *vata* person hardly sweats at all, even when the weather is hot. They seem to need to absorb heat and there is little activity in the sweat glands directed to reducing body temperature. The handshake is always dry and usually cool. The high metabolic rate in *pitta* people means they may have a need to lose excess body heat, to keep their temperature normal, even when the weather is cold. These are people who are always sweating; the handshake is slightly damp, though generally hot as well. For *kapha*, the tendency to sweat is average; the handshake may be slightly damp, though rather cooler than in the case of a *pitta* person.

Please mark the feature that *best* describes you.

SWEAT			
Characteristic:	*Vata*	*Pitta*	*Kapha*
Sweat	❏ Little	❏ Much	❏ Moderate

MOUTH AND LIPS

In keeping with the nature of *vata*, the jaw is either too small or too large so that the teeth do not fit in the mouth evenly. There is often great variability in the size of individual teeth and, like the nails, they are rather brittle, with thin enamel. There is an increased sensitivity of the teeth to cold and hot. The tongue is frequently thinly coated. (Be careful because the tongue is easily affected by your current nature, *vikruti*, and just by looking at it in a mirror may be misleading with regard to your *prakruti*.) The lips are thin, occasionally almost nonexistent.

Pitta mouths have regular jaws, even teeth of medium size that fit together well. High metabolic activity means cavities frequently occur in these teeth unless they are kept scrupulously clean. The gums are soft and reddish and the teeth tend to be yellowish. The tongue is often coated but frequently appears red and may even seem inflamed. The lips are clearly defined and on the full-colored, red side.

Lucky *kapha* individuals have large, evenly sized, strong white teeth that are generally resistant to disease. The tongue is seldom coated, but if it is, it tends to be thick and white. Their lips are very full — fuller than *pitta* lips though perhaps not as well defined — and always moist.

Please mark the features that *best* describe you.

MOUTH AND LIPS			
Characteristic:	Vata	Pitta	Kapha
Teeth	❏ Uneven/ crooked	❏ Regular/ off white	❏ Regular/ white
Lips	❏ Thin	❏ Well-defined, of moderate thickness	❏ Full and moist

APPETITE

Vata individuals are always "hungry," but since their eyes are often larger than their stomachs their appetites are soon satisfied. The appetite varies from day to day and from meal to meal, in accordance with the character of vata. These constitutions often "need" to eat between meals to prevent tiredness or dizziness.

People with *pitta* featuring strongly in their constitution have robust appetites and always enjoy eating. The desire for food is less variable than the *vata* person's and while there is less tendency to eat between meals, these people dislike missing meals or changing the time when they eat.

Kapha people have regular appetites, usually moderate, though they may eat at times just to fill their time. They are able to fast without any problem because they have so much energy stored as fat.

Please mark the feature that *best* describes you.

APPETITE			
Characteristic:	*Vata*	*Pitta*	*Kapha*
Appetite"	❏ Erratic, constantly eating, but soon "full"	❏ Strong/ excessive, need regular meals	❏ Steady, can go without eating

THIRST

One day *vata* types will be constantly thirsty and it may seem that no matter how much they drink their thirst cannot be quenched. Much of this desire is, however, in the mind and typically these are people who get a drink and then later find the glass half finished.

Pitta people tend to be excessively thirsty. They need to drink regularly and become very thirsty if they miss a routine drink at a particular time of the day.

Kapha individuals never really feel thirsty, unless they are perspiring a lot. Their mouths are always moist and they leave drinks unconsumed, not so much because the desire is in the mind more than the body, but because they simply do not feel particularly thirsty.

Please mark the feature that *best* describes you.

THIRST			
Characteristic:	*Vata*	*Pitta*	*Kapha*
Thirst	❑ Variable, lots of drinks half consumed	❑ Always drinking	❑ Low

BOWEL MOVEMENTS

In health, the bowels move once or twice a day without the need of laxatives or hard effort. If your bowels do not move once a day with occasional rare exceptions, then you are suffering from constipation. If the bowels move three or more times a day and the stool is loose then diarrhea is present.

Many people believe that the passed stool is the residue of undigested food and is absorbed in the small intestine; in health, this is not true. The stool consists mainly of dead cells from the lining of the intestine (they are all totally replaced every couple of days), together with dead bacteria from the colon. These bacteria are extremely important to the health of the entire intestine; they are critical for the digestion of certain food substances that enter the large bowel (mainly soluble fiber, not to be confused with insoluble fiber such as bran). They convert this special form of soluble fiber into substances that are essential for the nutrition of the tissues in the intestine itself. They are the digestive fire of the large bowel. Like the cells of the gut lining, which turn over rapidly and therefore need constant nutrition to be recreated, they have a limited life and must be excreted regularly. Indeed, if a person fasts, the weight of the stool changes very little from when they are eating. If food particles are present in the stool, then the fire in either the large or the small bowel, or both, is probably inadequate.

Vata people frequently complain about constipation; the stools tend to be hard, dark and difficult to pass; they often suffer often from gas and at times may become bloated or experience gurgling noises in the abdomen. In common with the other characteristics of *vata* types, they may experience variability, with spells of diarrhea in between periods of constipation. *Vata* people know that occasionally they have to use dietary adjustments to normalize their bowel habits, or even resort to strong laxatives.

The *pitta* person is one whose bowel habits are as regular as clockwork. The stools are usually well formed, but can be loose at times and may cause a burning sensation following a spicy meal.

Regular bowel movements once a day are characteristic of a *kapha* constitution. The stools are routinely well formed.

Please mark the feature that *best* describes you.

Bowel Movements			
Characteristic:	*Vata*	*Pitta*	*Kapha*
Bowel Movements"	❑ Gassy, erratic, hard and dry with bouts of constipation	❑ Regular, occasionally loose	❑ Heavy, bulky, often sinks

SEX DRIVE

The sex drive or libido of the *vata* person is extremely varied from day to day; it can be affected by fantasies and can appear to be "all or nothing." Excessive expenditure of effort in sexual intercourse leaves the *vata* person tired, owing to a lack of stored energy.

Strong, passionate sexual desire typifies the *pitta* personality. Passion is readily aroused and fulfilled if possible. The *pitta* person, frequently being the one to initiate intercourse, takes control of it. Being clear about what they want tends to mean they become upset if they do not achieve it.

Once again, the *kapha* individual demonstrates stability, loyalty, staying power and balance. They are almost never as intense as the *pitta* type and are slow to become aroused; however, once stimulated, their sexual energy declines very slowly.

Please mark the feature that *best* describes you.

SEX DRIVE			
Characteristic:	*Vata*	*Pitta*	*Kapha*
Libido	❏ Variable — all or nothing	❏ Passionate, domineering	❏ Steady, loyal, slow but sustained

MENSTRUATION

Menstruation can be the most difficult aspect of body function to assess because every woman's view of what is normal or heavy is colored by her experience over the years. The *vata* woman may experience a period that is heavy for her, but which a *pitta* woman would regard as light.

Women with a *vata* constitution frequently have very irregular cycles; they classically miss periods when exercising too much or eating insufficiently. Periods are often late, but can be early as well. The flow is variable, sometimes scanty and sometimes with clots. The flow is often dark in color. Sometimes they experience constipation and abdominal cramping a few days before their period actually starts.

Women with a *pitta* constitution usually have reliably regular cycles, but the flow tends to be for five or six days and can be quite heavy. It is bright red and cramps can be quite troublesome.

Women with a *kapha* constitution have regular periods, with relatively little experience of cramping, but they do tend to be troubled by water retention manifested often by a marked feeling of fullness in the breasts.

Please mark the feature that *best* describes you.

MENSTRUATION			
Characteristic:	*Vata*	*Pitta*	*Kapha*
Menstruation	❏ Variable, scanty, erratic	❏ Regular, heavy with cramps	❏ Regular, with premenstrual water reten- tion

PULSE

First introduced in the thirteenth century A.D., the pulse is a very important part of ayurvedic diagnosis. It is a complex and acquired skill to be able to assess the balance of the doshas from the nature of the pulse and is best performed by an ayurvedic physician. It is possible to discern the *prak-ruti* and also the *vikruti*, but this is an art that requires many years of patient practice. You can, though, check certain aspects of your own pulse. (It should preferably be tested first thing in the morning before breakfast.)

Sit quietly for five or ten minutes, away from any source of direct heat, and breathe quietly. Turn the right hand palm upward and wrap the second, third and fourth fingers of the left hand under the right wrist until they are resting on top of the wrist, just in line with the second finger of that hand, two fingers' width from the hand itself. Press gently with the finger tips and you will be able to feel the radial pulse. Now decrease the pressure of your fingers tips slightly and take note of the characteristics of the throbbing beat of the pulse. Your index or second finger denotes the *vata dosha*, the middle finger the *pitta dosha* and the ring finger the *kapha dosha*. The strongest pulse is the *dosha* that is predominant in the body. The doshas are also responsible for the nature of the pulse itself: *vata* controls the rhythm/regularity, *pitta* determines the speed and *kapha* the volume.

The *vata* pulse is thin and thready, often with a rhythm that varies markedly as you breathe — it may even be highly ir-regular. When *vata* predominates, the pulse appears to move in waves like a snake. The pulse of a purely *pitta* person is regular and strong, about seventy beats per minute, and varies only slightly as you breathe; it is said to "jump" like a frog. A *kapha* pulse is powerful, full, slow and regular; it is likened to the swimming of a swan.

Please mark the features that *best* describe you.

PULSE			
Characteristic:	*Vata*	*Pitta*	*Kapha*
Strongest pulse located under	❏ Index finger	❏ Middle finger	❏ Ring finger
Nature	❏ Feeble, irregular, 90 per minute	❏ Regular, prominent 70-80 per minute	❏ Full, steady, 60-70 per minute

SPEECH

Vata people are able to speak about almost anything. Often, however, they may find themselves talking about something completely different from what they started off with. Their voices tend to be breathy, and they love speaking, especially with another *vata* person, for hours on end.

If *pitta* is your constitution, the precision and fire of your make up will come through in your voice. You know what you want to say and the sort of response you expect from the listener. Your tone may carry impatience in it and you will often feel impatient to say what you wish to communicate. Conversations with another *pitta* individual tend to develop into arguments, or at least heated discussions. You are someone who speaks your mind — often regardless of the consequences.

Slow and measured speech is the hallmark of the *kapha* person. You think carefully about what you say and don't give too much away. You may be reticent to communicate. What you do say is important and is conveyed with weight, using a mellifluous tone of voice. When talking with another *kapha* person, there tend to be large gaps in the conversation that cause no discomfort to either party. This contrasts with the *pitta* individual, who feels the opportunity has come to pour out what he has been burning to say; and with the *vata*, who feels he must fill the silence with anything, relevant or not.

Please mark the feature that *best* describes you.

SPEECH			
Characteristic:	*Vata*	*Pitta*	*Kapha*
Speech	❏ Fast, high pitched, changing from one subject to another	❏ Intense, and incisive; loves debate	❏ Slow and measured, low pitched

PHYSICAL ACTIVITY

Vata people are very active and frequently restless; always on the move, they fidget constantly but with little staying power. Their appetite is driven to a large extent by their most recent physical activity; hard work makes them hungry. Their coordination is often poor and they are prone to sudden bursts of activity that achieve no particular purpose. Activities can be left uncompleted through lack of stamina. *Vata* people relish frequent hard exercise because of addiction to the internal morphinelike substances (endorphins) released by the body in response to exertion.

Individuals with a *pitta* make up can sustain prolonged hard exercise, but it tends to make them feel rather hot. Such exercise increases their thirst as much as their appetites. These are competitive people who often love sports.

A *kapha* constitution is exemplified by lethargy; *kaphas* do not generally wish to exercise, although if they do, it does not affect the appetite, which tends to be constant. High energy expenditure causes sweating, though at a moderate pace it may seem they can go on forever without difficulty; sudden bursts of extreme energy are not their style.

Please mark the feature that *best* describes you.

PHYSICAL ACTIVITY			
Characteristic:	Vata	Pitta	Kapha
Activity	❏ Very active, tends to fidget, expends energy quickly with poor endurance	❏ Moderately active, generally has lots of energy — likes sports and has desire to win	❏ Lethargic, slow moving but with excellent stamina and coordination

SLEEP

Vata people wake from sleep easily and tend to sleep restlessly. Their sleep patterns are, predictably, variable. They often grind their teeth at night and not infrequently sleep-talk; the mind is still active, even though they are supposed to be resting. They awake in the morning often feeling unrested.

Pitta people fall asleep readily, sleep lightly and wake up ready to take on the new day. If they should wake up during the night they go back to sleep without any difficulty.

Kaphas rapidly fall into slumber while reading or listening to music; they sleep deeply and are seldom roused during the night. Sleep comes easily at any time of day or night.

Please mark the feature that *best* describes you.

SLEEP			
Characteristic:	Vata	Pitta	Kapha
Sleep	❏ Light, fitful, unrefreshing, sleep talking	❏ Easy, short, refreshing	❏ Heavy, prolonged, slow to wake

DREAMING

People with a *vata* constitution dream profusely, or at least are aware of their dreams because they wake so frequently; by the time morning comes, however, they have forgotten what the dreams were about. Dreams are usually filled with activity. Motion is common, especially the sensation of being able to fly.

Pitta dreams are also intense, frequently passionate, and can be remembered the next day, at least for a while. *Pitta* dreams are frequently in color; particularly vivid colors can be recalled later, with an intensity that is typical of the *pitta* constitution.

Kapha in the constitution causes emotional rather than passionate dreams. Frequently they are calm, relaxed, matter-of-fact dreams of situations rather than any sensation of movement.

Please mark the feature that *best* describes you.

DREAMING			
Characteristic:	*Vata*	*Pitta*	*Kapha*
Dreams"	❏ Filled with activity, easily forgotten	❏ Passionate, in color, remembered	❏ Relaxed, emotional, not easily remembered

EMOTIONAL TEMPERAMENT

This aspect of your nature is related to how you react when facing a difficult situation. This is how you feel under these circumstances, not necessarily the emotional response that you display; you may have been taught to react in defined ways, but this seldom affects how you actually feel.

Vata people show fear and anxiety as a first reaction to any potentially threatening situation outside their control. If you are of this type, then you experience a dry mouth and a degree of panic. Thoughts will fly around your mind in a chaotic jumble.

Pitta is fire, which tends to ignite passionate feelings such as anger, or a clear response, knowing exactly what to do for the best. Your thoughts are ordered and logical and your response straightforward and precise.

If you are a *kapha* person you stay away from stressful situations because you do not like change. This may be such a strong trait that you bury your head in the sand rather than face the circumstances. Sometimes the situation does go away, but if not, then your emotional response tends to build up inside and may seriously accumulate over time. This can result, paradoxically, in unexpected occasional reactions.

Please mark the feature that *best* describes you.

EMOTIONAL TEMPERAMENT			
Characteristic:	*Vata*	*Pitta*	*Kapha*
Emotion"	❑ Anxious, insecure and unpredictable	❑ Forceful, irritable and jealous	❑ Calm but attached

CREATIVITY

There is a constant movement of ideas in the mind of the *vata* individual. A readiness to connect the apparently unconnected leads to great creativity. New ideas springing from the old make these people excellent at coming up with new theories, which may be seen by some as "crazy." As for implementing or testing new ideas, their tendency to be changeable and their inability to focus means this is best left to the other types.

Pitta characters are excellent at the first stage of implementing a new idea. They have the passion to make sure the idea works. Their creativity is in the realm of modifying an original idea so that it works in practice. Once they have achieved this goal though, they will then move on to the next idea. It is very much the "doing" that is important to them. The organization of a project or dealing with the day-to-day detail is best left to a *kapha* person.

Kaphas have both feet on the ground. They have the tenacity to polish something until it positively shines. This is equally creative, but at the opposite end of the spectrum from the *vata* type. *Kaphas* are brilliant organizers, although occasionally their determination can lead to inflexibility.

Please mark the feature that *best* describes you.

CREATIVITY			
Characteristic:	*Vata*	*Pitta*	*Kapha*
Creativity	❑ New ideas, flashes of inspiration	❑ Practical, molding, developing ideas and making them work	❑ Polishing, refining, good at organizing others

MEMORY

Short memories are characteristic of *vata* people. They seldom hold grudges — they simply can't remember long enough to be able to. What happened recently can be remembered extremely well, but remote memory is almost nonexistent.

The *pitta* memory is sharp — these people remember easily and do not readily forget.

Kapha individuals find it difficult to remember something and need to hear or experience it more than once before it becomes fixed in the mind. However, "once remembered, never forgotten" is the motto that applies to them.

Please mark the feature that *best* describes you.

MEMORY			
Characteristic:	*Vata*	*Pitta*	*Kapha*
Memory	❑ Recent memory good, past memory poor	❑ Very sharp	❑ Slow to commit to memory, but never forgets

PERSONALITY

Vata people are highly susceptible to external influences and react quickly to changes in their circumstances. Change in all things at all times is typical; one minute they desire company and a moment later need solitude. It can be difficult to keep up with their changeable moods, one minute ecstatic, the next depressed. Friendships come and go. They seem unwilling to adopt any pattern in their daily existence to the extent that they seldom finish what they start. If motivated, they can be the driving force behind anything, the life and soul of the party, but will seldom be there at the end. Many of their decisions and emotions arise from feelings of uncertainty.

Pragmatic, clear and powerful in their actions and emotions, *pitta* characters can become domineering. They are always passionate and thus intrinsically brave but well balanced. This passionate nature leads to reliable enthusiasm and commitment, but can be negative if something makes them angry. They can be equally committed to wreaking vengeance in a sharp and hurtful way. Everything has a purpose, including their friendships. Passion may run so high that they are intolerant of anyone who gets in their way, not hesitating to "burn" them if it suits their purpose.

Kapha individuals are, on the whole, calm, peaceful and reliable people who are most at ease in the cozy environment of home and family. Unfortunately, some of these characteristics may lead, in excess, to idleness, addiction, jealousy and selfishness. However, these people usually have personalities that are rock solid, so stable that they may appear to be inactive in both mind and body. They usually take an inordinate amount of time to start an activity but will see it through to the end with stubborn determination regardless of difficulties. This aspect is true of every branch of their lives; friendships form slowly but persist to the grave.

Please mark the feature that *best* describes you.

PERSONALITY			
Characteristic:	*Vata*	*Pitta*	*Kapha*
Personality	❏ Uncertain, changeable, short relationships	❏ Passionate, brave, purposeful relationships	❏ Calm, reliable, stubborn, lasting relationships

ORGANIZATION AND DAILY ROUTINE

Vata characters are the antithesis of creatures of habit. They never keep good records and money-wise are always in a mess. The normal routines of life such as eating, drinking and sleeping happen with little apparent pattern except that imposed by society and circumstance. Their houses are generally disorganized, with the things they might need tomorrow left out "just in case."

Pitta people are the planners and organizers of this world. They are financially well organized, work out what they can afford to spend and do it very sensibly. They are not creatures of habit, but use their habits for their own ends, modifying them as they go along. Their homes are neat and tidy in a purposeful way — they know where everything is and why.

Kapha people are almost exclusively creatures of habit. They revel in habits to the point that they often get stuck in a groove like a record on an old gramophone. They are financially prudent and always have resources put away for a rainy day. When taken to extremes they may appear to spend little and infrequently. Their homes are a picture of compulsive neatness. Nothing is thrown away; everything is stored in case it is needed one day.

Please mark the features that *best* describe you.

ORGANIZATION AND DAILY ROUTINE			
Characteristic:	*Vata*	*Pitta*	*Kapha*
Organization"	❏ Disorganized, difficulty sticking to routines	❏ Neat, tidy and purposeful	❏ Very neat, storing everything away for a rainy day
Finances"	❏ Impulse buying, financial chaos	❏ Clear financial planning, purposeful buying	❏ Saver, tends not to spend

SUMMARIES OF CONSTITUTIONAL TYPES

Add up the number of marks you have for each of the categories *vata*, *pitta* and *kapha* in answering the questions above. Usually one or two types will have a higher total than the others. These higher totals indicate what sort of basic constitution you have — your *prakruti*. For example, if you counted approximately twelve *vatas*/twenty-four *pittas*/four *kaphas*, your basic constitution is probably predominately *pitta* with an element of *vata* (*pitta-vata*). If you counted three *vatas*/thirty-four *pittas*/three *kaphas*, your constitution is predominately *pitta*. If there is an even balance between the three doshas, then add up again but using only those marks with a """ beside them. This should give you a clear view of the balance of the doshas in your constitution.

Below are summaries, in general terms, of the various constitutional types. No account has been taken for the predominance of one characteristic over another when two doshas predominate over the third. For example, twelve *vatas*, twenty-four *pittas*, four *kaphas* and twenty-four *vatas*, twelve *pittas*, four *kaphas* both represent *pitta-vata* constitutions and are dealt with by a single summary.

However, in the former case there will be a tendency toward *pitta* and thus the *pitta* summary should be read as well; and in the latter case there will be a tendency toward *vata*, in which case understanding will be helped by reading the *vata* summary in combination with *pitta-vata*. Listed first are the simple types where one dosha is much more evident than the other two and then the mixtures (most of us) are listed where one dosha is clearly much less evident than the other two.

VATA

Vata people are usually rather thin and do not gain weight easily except when they overindulge in food. They have narrow shoulders and hips and their joints tend to make cracking noises when flexed. They find it hard to sit still. They have dry, rough skin that chaps easily and is prone to corns and calluses. Similarly, their hair tends to be coarse, dry and curly. They suffer from the cold and frequently complain of poor circulation in the extremities. The skin is often cool to the touch, they sweat little and enjoy a warm climate, preferably full sunlight.

The appetite is unpredictable; it is easily affected by overindulgence in activities that are exciting or absorbing to the point that eating is forgotten, sometimes resulting in further damage to the digestion. Dietary preferences are akin to the love of certain types of weather — *vatas* adore hot food.

Their ability to do things is variable, due to extreme fluctuations of their energy levels related to their irregular eating and sleeping habits. The *vata* person keeps going, despite needing to take a rest, by consuming large quantities of tea and coffee. Not recognizing that this leads to continued frenetic activity followed by exhaustion reinforces the pattern of life that typifies the *vata* individual. Despite the tendency to reach the stage of utter fatigue, they often have difficulty falling asleep, or once asleep they continually wake and fall asleep, often oversleeping in the morning. They can reach such a level of exhaustion that they sleep as if comatose.

Sensations tend to be excessively appreciated; they are typically nervous and jumpy. The sound of a door slamming will cause them to jump out of their skins and they may overreact to painful stimuli. The need to reduce this type of overstimulation may express itself in the *vata* person as fear. Soothing music, soft oily massage and a quiet, warm environment without extremes are what these people prefer.

The lack of habitual routines in life leads to chaos in their lifestyle. If absence of control and peace typifies your life, then you almost certainly have *vata* as your key predominant dosha.

PITTA

Pitta people are well built and well proportioned. They have regular, hearty appetites and their eating habits are well planned. Weight can be gained if there is overeating, but this is unusual. They are intense people, sometimes to the extent of being seen as sharp, irritable or intolerant. Red, the color of fire, characterizes these individuals, resulting in fair skin, often with freckles and moles. They blush easily and also burn readily in the sun, which tends to amplify the freckles. The hair is generally straight, fair or red in color. Indeed, anyone who has red hair has *pitta* as a significant element of their *prakruti*. They sweat readily because of all the heat stored inside.

Pittas have razor-sharp minds and are usually witty. Because of this and the hot, intense nature of fire, they do not tolerate fools easily. They tend toward impatience. They usually sleep soundly because it is part of their "plan." They apply the same passion and ambition to all they do, at work or play. They will see a task through to its end with a purposeful approach. *Pitta* types prefer cool, well-structured environments.

KAPHA

The *kapha* person is normally large framed with natural athletic skills, especially while at school. The problem, however, tends to be that they gain weight just by looking at food, especially if not exercising. This leads to a loss of athletic ability as the years go by. The majority of people with a *kapha* constitution are healthy most of the time, but overeating may cause illness, which is out of character with their nature.

Kaphas have heavy emotional needs and frequently fulfill them by using food as a substitute. Their innate feeling of hunger, however, is never as intense as that of the *pitta* person, and is always more regular than that of the *vata* individual. It is a *kapha's* need for emotional satisfaction that modifies his or her appetite and leads to a paradoxically high appetite. *Kapha* people are often a serious mix of paradoxes. They sleep very soundly and have a natural tendency to oversleep.

They are laidback people who, on the whole, do not hunger for the same degree of excitement and arousal that *vata* and *pitta* people love. Once aroused, however, their appetites — for sex, for example — may become very strong. They are slow to rouse, but then their athletic nature breaks through and maintains their drive to reach the end. *Kapha* people are stable, outwardly somewhat slow, and may appear to be complacent. They are creatures of habit and may become stuck in a rut because the environment they have is so enjoyable that they resist change and may become greedy, obdurate or overtly reactionary.

DUAL CONSTITUTIONS

If you have just one predominant dosha, you know how you are going to react to any situation. However, if you have more than one, you can never be absolutely sure which dosha is going to be the most influential in any given circumstance. In one situation, one dosha will be important in gauging your response, in another situation it will be the alternative. These constitutions are mixtures of *vata* and *pitta*, *kapha* and *pitta* or *vata* and *kapha* and you will probably fit into one of these categories. The examples below are very general, and cannot take account of the fact that as an individual you will probably have a somewhat different balance than the example quoted — so do not expect a complete match.

Vata-Pitta (or Pitta-Vata)

These people often have the cold hands and feet that are the bane of the *vata* individual's life. They also love warm climates, despite the *pitta* element in their make-up. The *pitta* influence, however, does limit the degree of heat they feel comfortable with. They love to eat but have great difficulty in digesting food properly, especially raw food.

In many areas of the outward signs of their constitution they show combined characteristics. For example, the combination of the curly hair of the *vata* character and the straight hair of the *pitta* individual leads frequently to wavy hair. More frequently, the effects of *vata* and *pitta* appear predominately in different areas of the individual. Furthermore, the two doshas can alternate with each other depending upon the circumstances. Thus a *vata-pitta* type may feel insecure in one confrontational situation and yet on another day experience severe anger at the same type of situation; it depends upon the balance within the person at the time. Worst of all, both may be present almost simultaneously so that the person knows what to do to solve a particular problem, but then feels insecure about the ability to actually do it.

This duality can, nonetheless, be the *vata-pitta* person's greatest asset if properly directed. Imagine the *vata* ability for original thought and spontaneity, combined with the passion and application of *pitta*. It is a combination that is without equal, but it needs proper direction. Without balance it can lead to frenetic attachment to sensual pleasure as the source of fulfillment; it is the opportunity for development of self-awareness that must be explored, for this will create the stability that this character-type so desperately needs.

Pitta-Kapha (or Kapha-Pitta)

The combination of the *kapha*'s stability together with *pitta*'s ability to accommodate change results in a personality that is perhaps more capable than most in coping with our turbulent world. There is, of course, a downside that is a combination of the self-satisfied smugness of the *kapha* individual together with the superior and egotistical nature of the *pitta* person. These people can become wrapped up in their own little world to the total exclusion of others — they can be impossible to live with!

However, they are often successful people. The power and enthusiasm of the *pitta* is expressed superbly in *kapha*'s solid physique; the balance of emotions is such that they are slow to anger, unlike pure *pittas*, but do not store emotions for too long, unlike the pure *kapha*. Climate is of little concern to them because they have the ability to cope with both extremes of hot and cold.

Owing to their low inherent *vata*, *pitta-kapha* types need to achieve balance by spiritual exploration and discipline. They also need to be "kicked" by unusual situations occasionally in order to prevent the smug overconfidence that can be their hallmark.

Vata-Kapha (or Kapha-Vata)

This combination can be the most difficult to deal with because of the extreme opposite nature of the two doshas involved. The doshas do have one thing in common, a propensity for coldness — they lack fire. The insulating qualities of *kapha* tend to prevent this as a perceived symptom. The difficulties that arise do so because of the lack of fire more than anything else. This low fire (or *agni*) means they tend to have digestive problems. They are not able to digest food fully and so the bowel itself will be poorly nourished, leading to gassy indigestion and frequent bouts of constipation mixed with occasional diarrhea. The other important area affected by the lack of fire is in the emotional world. They have a very high level of need for emotional fire to be supplied by someone else.

Kapha-vata types are generally tall, but of average build. They do most things in earnest but sometimes make the *vata* mistake of not applying measure to their efforts. This can be most damaging when their emotional desires are frustrated; they impose a level of hurt upon themselves that is located very deeply and tends never to be forgotten. It is a feature of the indiscretion of the *vata* and elephantine memory of the *kapha*.

They are excellent examples of the potential for alternation of characteristics in people ruled by two doshas. They can be fancy-free one minute, yet profound and secretive the next.

THE MEANING OF YOUR *PRAKRUTI*

You should not view the above analysis as an attempt to fit you and your constitution into a box — nothing could be further from the truth. The concept of constitutional types is basically straightforward, though it may not seem so right now. It will become clearer as you observe the way you live in this world. We all have a body and mind quite unlike that of any other person, although ultimately the central light within us all that is our "self" *is* identical. It is simply the body and mind which differ from person to person and that need to be kept in balance to achieve perfect health. The exercise of finding out which constitutional type you are does not bind you to one stereotype; it provides you with information on qualities which are so deeply intrinsic in you that they must be consciously balanced. It provides a simple foundation on which you can work to create a new, balanced healthy you.

Remember that your assessment of your constitution is affected to some extent by that very constitution. This is not a problem — it simply means that some of your perceptions of yourself may not be absolutely accurate at the moment. As you come into a better state of balance within yourself, it will become more apparent what the accurate answers are. It is important to revisit this chapter perhaps every three months to reassess your *prakruti*. Try to do this as if for the first time; it will not be easy, but you will reap the rewards in the long run.

6

TREATMENT WITH AYURVEDA

According to ayurvedic teaching, starting any form of treatment without first dealing with the toxins in the system that have caused the disease will only make matters worse. In the short term, treatment may superficially relieve the symptoms, but the imbalance in the doshas will manifest as disease again either in the same location or elsewhere. Toxins may either be eliminated or neutralized. This applies to both the physical and emotional level of disease.

THE EMOTIONAL LEVEL

Anxiety, anger, fear, insecurity, jealousy and greed are human emotions recognized by us all, but as children we are taught that it is not appropriate to express these "negative" feelings. Ayurveda teaches us that this is incorrect thinking and that it is important to release these emotions otherwise imbalance in the doshas will occur, leading to a build up of disease-creating toxins.

First of all, we need to know what our repressed emotions are. Sometimes they have been so effectively buried that we are quite unaware of them. The only way to find out is through observation. This is a little more than plain observation of what is going on in our lives — it involves observing the observer, even though that sounds almost impossible. It helps to ask the question: "Who is it that observes you are happy (or sad or angry, etc.)?"; "Who is it that is aware you are seeing this page?" The answer is the true self, or the soul, unchangeable and unaffected by the exigencies of life; in Western medicine it is sometimes referred to as insight — literally looking inward.

There are many techniques to assist in this process of observation. It helps to pause for a couple of seconds before doing anything; discussion with a group of like-minded individuals refines the ability to make contact with this insight; meditation is extremely useful.

Observation is the key to understanding your emotions. For example, if anger arises, you should be completely aware of it — do not try to do anything about it, just observe it. In this way you will learn how it arose and what it resulted in. Release of anger is the important feature and, once again, this involves not doing anything; simple observation will enable its release.

THE PHYSICAL LEVEL

Diet

The guiding principle of Ayurveda is that each person has the power to heal herself. Much can be done to remove or neutralize toxins in the body by balancing the doshas, using an appropriate diet as part of a program of measure in all aspects of life. Such dietary adjustments also serve to maintain the balance of the doshas and thus perfect health. Spiritual development is vitally important, but it is difficult to maintain if the body and mind are ailing so our eating habits must be examined.

What is eaten should be chosen to balance the individual constitution. Choosing the proper diet is a simple matter when given an understanding of the constitution and how it relates to the qualities of various foods. The taste of the food (sweet, sour, salty, pungent, bitter or astringent) and the season of the year must also be considered.

You should not eat unless you are feeling hungry, nor drink unless you are feeling thirsty. Do not confuse these two feelings; it is a great temptation to drink in order to assuage hunger, but all that will happen is the digestive fire will be diluted.

In the process of eating you are feeding not just the body but the mind and spirit as well. It is important, therefore, to feed all five of the senses by preparing and consuming food that is attractive to look at, good to taste, inspiring to smell and pleasant in constitution. It may seem difficult to satisfy the sense of hearing but the sound of food being cooked or of a stick of raw celery being chewed can do so in a very pleasing way.

Always prepare, serve and eat food with love. We have all had the experience that food cooked by someone who loves us is somehow more pleasing than that cooked without love. To hold on to unloving feelings while we are eating tends to cause indigestion. Poor digestion will give rise to production of *ama* and thus to the promotion of disease. Drink water with your meal in sips. After you have finished eating, a mixture of yogurt and water will aid digestion. This drink should be about half yogurt and half water, but see what suits you best. If you have *vata* as a strong characteristic, then add a little lemon juice. If your major dosha is *pitta*, then add a little sugar. For *kapha* individuals, a little honey and a sprinkle of fresh black pepper is probably a good idea. This is specifically a drink for the end of, rather than during, a meal. The best drink during the meal itself is water; don't drink milk with a meal, especially if the food contains meat.

If possible, allow your food to pass through the digestive system before doing any strenuous exercise. When you exercise, the body reduces the blood supply to the gut and makes it available to the appropriate muscles; this disrupts the whole process of digestion and must be avoided if *ama* is not to be produced. The same is true of sleeping; the circulation of blood in the body changes profoundly and the gut is no longer supplied with what it needs to allow correct digestion and assimilation of what you have just eaten. Avoid both these "activities" for a good two hours after a meal. This does not mean that you cannot go for a stroll after eating — it is almost certainly beneficial to take a gentle walk following a meal.

Food has the property, as far as digestion is concerned, of being either heavy or light, related largely to the amount of digestion required. Light foods include cooked rice and potatoes, whereas heavy foods include things like raw food and cooked meat. In the West, we tend to think that salads are "light" food, but they actually require a lot more digestion than a cooked vegetable. Raw and cooked food have different amounts of *agni* present in them and should never be eaten in the same meal, except in very small quantities.

Light food makes it easier to integrate body, mind and spirit because there is less redistribution of blood to the gut for digestion. Heavy food always leaves you feeling tired and lethargic, and often actually induces sleep.

Diet and the Mind

Everything you eat will affect your mind as well as your body. In Ayurveda, the mind has three possible states that are related to the state of the constitution as a whole:

- *sattva*, or peaceful equilibrium, in which the power of discrimination is most accessible
- *rajas*, or activity, in which excessive thoughts prevent discrimination from being accessed

- *tamas*, or inertia, in which there is a heaviness and attachment to the physical realm such that there is neither activity nor discrimination.

This division of states of mind is the cause of another of those vicious circles that tend to characterize our lives. The power of discrimination allows us to know the correct balance and what is the most appropriate action in a certain situation. If this is clouded or access to it is not possible then we are unable to decide, for example, what to eat and how much; this can give rise to a more *tamasic* state, which further obscures discrimination!

Food that is bad, fermented or preserved for too long increases the amount of *tamas* in the body and then in the mind. A good example of a fermented food is alcohol. This does not mean we should not drink alcohol, but we are all aware of the effects of too much! Legumes and high-protein food like meat, fish and poultry increase *rajas*, as do any of the pungent spices. To increase *sattva* we should increase our intake of grains, fruits and most vegetables.

Dos and Don'ts

Always eat fresh foods when possible and avoid preserved, canned or frozen food items, though the latter are permissible if fresh is not available. Eat light foods until your appetite is satisfied, but do not be tempted to clear the plate just because there is food on it. With heavy foods, try to restrict yourself to satisfying only half your appetite with this type of ingredient. If you are ill, eat only light foods, and then in small quantities, until half your appetite — at the most — is fulfilled.

One of the most important rules in Ayurveda is never to combine in one meal foods that "fight," either in terms of the signals they give to the gut or in terms of their qualities:

- do not eat cooked foods and raw foods at the same meal since they require different types of digestion

- avoid combining heavy and light foods

- avoid drinking milk while eating radishes, tomatoes, potatoes, bananas, meat, fish, eggs, citrus fruits, melon, bread or cherries

- do not mix milk and yogurt

- eat fresh fruit separately from other meals (cooked fruit may be eaten at the same time as a cooked meal)

- avoid mixing different types of protein, such as meat and cheese.

In recent years, Western medical research has identified other unhelpful food combinations in line with the traditional ayurvedic ones above. Keep heavy high-protein or high-fat food items in separate meals from lighter foods such as starches and vegetables. These types of food require quite different digestive processes in the gut for proper nutrition. If you eat them together there will be competition for the appropriate digestive mechanism and neither will be digested properly. Proteins and fats require slow digestion and absorption by the small bowel, whereas starches need to pass quickly to the large bowel where they are acted upon by bacteria to produce special forms of nutrients. Your small bowel needs this form of food. If they are eaten together, then fat and protein slow down the passage of the starches and they do not reach the large bowel in time to be digested by this special bacterial mechanism. It is your bowel that suffers and is unable to function properly as the controller of nutrients entering the body.

Do your best to maintain the separations between different types of foods as indicated above — there is nothing "wrong" with any of them, they just do not combine well.

Taste

All foods have their own "taste" characteristics that interact with your body and your consciousness. These effects are complex and not necessarily obvious. Take a little piece of raw potato and chew it for four or five minutes. Observe the way that the taste changes as it is chewed; it begins by tasting rather dry and almost astringent, but after a while it starts to taste sweet. This is because it is being partly digested in your mouth, which makes it sweet tasting.

Understanding a particular food, taste, energy and post-digestive effect makes it easier to see how it is going to interact with your mind and body, but it can be difficult to remember all these influences. In appendices *Vata*, *Pitta* and *Kapha*, pages 90–104, you will find listed foods that may be eaten by people of various constitutions together with a list of those that should not be because of their tendency to aggravate the predominant *dosha* and create imbalance.

DUAL CONSTITUTIONS

If like most people you have two predominant doshas in your basic constitution, then read the following sections. You will by now have some idea which of the doshas in your mind and body are out of balance; you should apply the dietary rules appropriate for the dosha that is out of balance.

The following sections make reference to environmental factors, the chief among these being the effects of the seasons upon your present balance. Spring and summer are warm times, characterized by growth and activity. As a result, there is a natural increase of *pitta* in the constitutional balance and if this is your predominant dosha you will need to pay extra attention to keeping it under control. This applies equally to the other doshas; autumn is a time of increased *vata*, when winds are high, leaves are falling off the trees and everything is drying out. The depth of winter and the early part of spring are times when *kapha* is increased. We already tend to modify our diets naturally by eating salads in the summer and hot soup on a cold winter night.

VATA-PITTA

The external influences that affect your balance are the presence of increased *vata* in the environment in autumn and winter and excess *pitta* in the spring and summer. So as a general rule, you should follow the dietary advice for *vata* during autumn and winter, followed by the advice for *pitta* during the spring and summer. In each case, the dietary recommendations given in the appendices will help to keep each list's dosha under control.

Pungent tastes increase both *vata* and *pitta* doshas in the individual and the taste of sweet foods reduces both, so you should avoid spicy, pungent food however much you may be tempted. Try to keep your diet high in sweet items (sweet here means the ultimate effect of the taste, not necessarily the taste when you first put the food in your mouth).

PITTA-KAPHA

Because there are external environmental factors similar to those for the *vata-pitta* person affecting your mind and body, you should use the dietary advice given for *pitta* during the spring and summer, followed by the *kapha* dietary recommendations during autumn and winter. The food tastes you should avoid, because they aggravate both *pitta* and *kapha*, are sour and salty. The tastes that are good for you are essentially bitter and astringent.

VATA-KAPHA

As a result of external environmental factors affecting your mind and body, use the dietary advice for *vata* during the summer and autumn, together with that for *kapha* during the winter and spring months. Make sure that during the summer you have some sweet foods to help balance the *vata* and during the winter there are elements of bitter and astringent tastes to balance the *kapha*.

VATA INDIVIDUALS

Try to eat little and often; three or preferably four times a day. You may also eat snacks in between meals, but be sure to allow the previous meal to pass well into the digestive system before consuming the next one. Allow at least two hours between meals or snacks. If you eat more frequently your gut will still be in the appropriate state for digesting the previous food and will not be ready to start dealing with the next input.

You will do best with cooked food; keep raw food to a minimum and at all costs avoid fried foods. The variable nature of the digestion in *vata* people means that there is a particular problem with the digestive process if foods of markedly differing heaviness, or raw and cooked, are combined. The gut needs a clear signal as to which type of food it is going to be dealing with or it becomes confused and agitated. This is why separating raw and cooked food is much more important for pure *vata* types than for others.

The *vata* person's diet should also be as regular as possible since irregularity will aggravate *vata* and add to the problem of poor digestion. It should be as balanced as possible, with no excess of any particular food type because *vata* is always aggravated by excess. Try to avoid foods that have bitter, pungent or astringent tastes.

Any sweetener may be used sparingly in food preparation, although white sugar should never be used. Avoid bread that has been made with yeast because the gassy nature of the yeast will increase *vata*; however, as all bread is somewhat dry and has some sort of gas-producing mechanism in its production, it should only be eaten in moderation.

All vegetables must be cooked and those on the list to be avoided (See Appendix *Vata*) are permissible to eat if cooked and not consumed too frequently. If you feel like an occasional salad make sure it is covered with plenty of sweet, oily dressing. Fruits permitted for the *vata* individual must never be eaten in a dried form (for example, dried apricots). Eat them stewed or fresh occasionally. Avoid fruit that is unripe — it tends to be astringent, especially bananas.

You can benefit from a small amount of meat in your diet, but see the list for recommended and prohibited meats. Excessive meat consumption will weaken your digestion, though in small quantities it is useful because it provides a complete protein balance, plus has a "grounding" effect.

All beans should be eaten in moderation because they are high in protein and will lead to an increase of gaseous nitrogenous waste products if consumed in excess. The *vata* nature of these proteins can be reduced to some extent by soaking them and discarding the water before cooking; cooking them in fresh water. The presence of ginger or garlic when cooking beans can increase *agni* and reduce the gas-producing tendency, as can adding a little oil. It is best to experiment and see what technique produces the least gas in the intestine.

Provided you do not have a dairy allergy, dairy products are good for you — with the proviso that hard cheeses should be eaten sparingly.

Vata people often like hot spices, but beware of their tendency to aggravate *vata* in the long run. Also, if you have a significant element of *pitta* in your constitution then the spices will be disastrous in their effect on the *pitta* dosha. Your naturally addictive personality will strongly crave nicotine, white sugar and caffeine if exposed to them; avoid them at all costs. Alcohol in moderation is of benefit to the *vata* person, but "moderation" is the key word.

PITTA INDIVIDUALS

You should eat three well-defined meals per day, with a gap of at least four and preferably six hours between them. You may have snacks, but leave a gap of three hours between your meals and your snacks. Avoid fried foods because the process of frying adds intense heat to the food and this can destabilize *pitta*. Raw foods are good for you and your digestion has enough *agni* to be able to deal with them. Cooked foods will tend to increase *pitta* too much if you are not careful.

Avoid hot tastes — sour, salty or pungent — in your food and place emphasis in your diet on the sweet, bitter and astringent tastes. Specific foods to avoid are: meat, eggs, salt and alcohol. Vegetables, grain and fruit as listed in the "Appendix *Pitta*" are the best foods for you. Yours should be a largely vegetarian diet; however, there are a few meats listed in the appendix that can be eaten infrequently and in small quantity without doing too much harm.

Avoid bread that has been made with yeast because of the sour nature of the fermentation process. Nonyeast or unleavened breads are excellent for you. Vegetables can be eaten raw, and should be consumed frequently. However, avoid hot vegetables such as radishes and peppers. Generally red vegetables — for example, tomatoes — are forbidden.

Remember to select fruit that is sweet and avoid those that are sour — this may apply simply to how ripe something is, so do not eat a fruit on the recommended list if it is unripe. Citrus fruits in small quantities reduce *pitta* because their post-digestive effect is not heating unless consumed in large quantities. This is because the acid in them is capable of being removed easily from the body via the lungs as carbon dioxide, thus leaving anti-*pitta* residue.

Meat should be avoided, especially seafood, which is said to be "hot" and can cause allergies. Egg yolks are hot and egg whites cooling, so eggs need to be separated into their component parts and the yolk thrown away most of the time! You have the luxury of being able to digest almost anything, but beware of a large quantity of beans; the same waste products that affect *vata* individuals so badly also aggravate the *pitta* dosha.

If you eat a vegetarian diet be careful to avoid nuts and oils in general. These are too heating for the *pitta* person with one or two exceptions, such as coconut, which has a very cooling effect. All dairy products — milk, unsalted butter, cream and soft cheese — are excellent. To avoid the negative tastes above, you should steer clear of hard cheeses, salted butter and yogurt, unless it has had some fire, such as cinnamon, added to it and has been diluted at least half and half with water. Any sweetener can be used (including white sugar) except molasses or honey, both of which are hot. Hot spices are guaranteed to increase the *pitta* part of your nature and a careful choice of cooling herbs should be made. The *pitta* individual should never add salt to her food.

KAPHA INDIVIDUALS

A *kapha* person should eat only two meals a day, allowing at least a six-hour gap between them. You should not take snacks in between. You will have a natural tendency to be able to eat as much as you feel like and so you must consciously make an effort to limit the total amount you eat at each meal. There is a relatively low amount of digestive fire, or *agni*, and you should generally stick to cooked food. Occasional consumption of raw foods will help to clean the intestine, but overindulgence will cause digestive problems because of the lack of intrinsic fire. As for the other doshas, fried foods should always be avoided because the heaviness of the fat will tend to aggravate the *kapha* dosha.

You need to pay attention in your diet to bitter, pungent and astringent foods. You need to avoid the sweet, sour and salty food elements and you should stay clear of dairy products altogether. If you wish to eat grains or bread make sure the grains are roasted or the bread is toasted. You need "heat" in your foods and the grains listed in the "Appendix *Kapha*" have been selected with this in mind. Different types of grain have different amounts of intrinsic heat within them; wheat, for instance, is very heavy, oily and cold, and should therefore be avoided.

All vegetables are good for you, with the exception of potatoes, tomatoes and water chestnuts. You can eat as many vegetables as often as you like, but remember not to have them raw except on occasion. Root vegetables tend to be sweet, and thus should take second place to those growing above ground. The fruits you eat should be "dry," like apples, and not those that are full of water or that are very sweet or very sour.

Try to stay away from meat, but if you feel the need to eat it make sure it is dry-roasted or grilled; never have fried meat — you do not need its grounding effect. Stick to the list recommended in the "Appendix *Kapha*." The same principles apply to the various beans that are available; you do not need very much of them so restrict your intake and stay away from the heavier varieties such as kidney beans. If you do have beans, eat them in small quantities.

Nuts and seeds contain large amounts of oils and are definitely not for you. In fact you should avoid oils of all sorts, as previously mentioned. This applies also to dairy products, which you should avoid. Under any circumstances do not use sweet substances of any sort.

Hot spices are an excellent idea in an attempt to increase the innate fire of the food you are eating. It is difficult for you to use too many!

YOUR WEIGHT
AND AYURVEDA

———

The world in which we live constantly urges us to consume. We are exhorted to lose weight by reducing the amount of fat and salt in our diets. Yet the food industry adds salt, sugar and fat to all processed foods, often to mask the poor taste of the ingredients or to create taste where none exists. There are other ways of adding flavor to prepared food but these are expensive. So it is hardly surprising that despite all the good intentions of weight-reduction programs aimed at improving our health, we are still becoming more and more overweight.

If you are of a predominantly *vata* constitution and you are overweight it is simply because you eat too much, or you may need to review your constitution to see if you have more *kapha* in your *prakruti* than you thought. *Pitta* people can gain weight easily, especially from overeating, but they also tend to be able to lose it readily.

7

If you have a *kapha* constitution there are two important things to be aware of: first, you will always have a well-rounded body (this does not mean obese) and you will never be able to — nor should you try to — achieve a thin, "super-model" image. Second, you will put on weight easily and tend to hang on to it.

This is also true for the *pitta-kapha* constitution. If you are *vata-pitta*, you will tend to have the same characteristic ability to gain and lose weight as the *pitta* individual. If you have *vata-kapha* characteristics, while you will find it difficult to lose weight, it also goes on quite slowly.

WHY ARE WE OVERWEIGHT?

We eat because we are told to; this was the case when we were children and now as adults through advertising. We also eat as a substitute for love, or as a way of trying to rectify imbalances in our doshas, especially on the emotional level — fear, insecurity, anger or depression. These imbalances are partially solvable by diet but it is more important to solve the problem that is causing the emotion in the first place. This latter aspect of treatment is in our own hands, but is not easy to approach and so it is important to seek professional help from an ayurvedic practitioner. Failing this, seek the support of your partner or best friend and listen to what they say. Try not to use food as a substitute.

Also, because processed foods are packed with salt, sugar and fat, make your own meals from fresh ingredients and do not use these additives. Do not buy processed foods or snacks, or even a ready-made sandwich unless it is labeled "no added salt" and "low fat." If you tend to buy snacks for lunch, try buying a freshly made sandwich so you can determine what goes into it — it is just about to go into *you*! Buy a banana, apple, orange or other fresh fruit, depending upon which are recommended in the list for your dosha.

DIETS

Simple calorie-controlled diets are inappropriate for modifying weight and yet many people are addicted to them. Reduced calorie intake is beneficial, but what is important is the *way* we reduce the calories and the reasons for doing so. Too often the desire to "go on a diet" represents a form of self-punishment because we feel guilty about our current body image. This is not a helpful attitude.

Crash diets usually represent a desire to lose weight rapidly. Remember that our weight and the ratio of fat in our bodies has built up over many years and expecting it to disappear in a few days or weeks is not realistic. If we starve ourselves (often the essential goal of a strict calorie-controlled diet) the weight will surely vanish; but by doing this we lose something called "lean body mass," the muscles and other tissues that make up the body and consume most of the calories we eat most of the time. If we lose lean body mass, when the diet stops we tend to return to what we were eating before and the weight goes back on faster than ever. This is because our energy expenditure, or basal metabolic rate (BMR), is now less than it was before the diet started because of the reduction in lean body mass.

Don't expect to lose more than one pound every week on average. In fact, you should only measure your weight once a week at the same time of the same day of the week, and even then only gauge whether you are actually losing weight once a month. This is because body weight varies naturally from one end of the day to the other and from day to day for all sorts of reasons, especially if you are a woman. One pound a week may not sound like very much — but think about it — that's 52 pounds in a year.

Exercise is usually recommended by anyone advising a weight-loss program, but why? The reasons are three-fold. Moderate exercise, such as a brisk walk for thirty minutes five times per week, preferably daily, will burn off a few calories. However, that is a relatively small effect — you won't notice any change in weight between the start and end of the walk!

Going for a brisk walk regularly has a much more important effect concerning the control of *vata*, which intrudes into the lives of all but a few of us. Analysis of our appetites shows that they vary from day to day between 2000 and 5000 calories, despite the fact that our energy expenditure is usually only about 2500 calories! This is a typical *vata* characteristic caused by our lifestyles. As energy expenditure by the individual increases towards 3500 calories, the top end of the appetite range comes down to 3500 calories, and from there on it goes up if energy expenditure goes up. Thus, the effect of exercise on the appetite can be quite dramatic. Even deep remedial massage can have a similar effect.

Exercise helps to maintain, or even increase lean body mass so that your basal metabolic rate goes up — meaning it is more difficult to put weight on again. That said, of course, you are not going to stop the diet you are on because in Ayurveda you will simply have changed the *way* you eat.

There is also evidence that exercising and losing weight alters something called insulin sensitivity. Insulin is the most important hormone in the body concerned with the control of calories. As we become overweight, it seems that the sensitivity of our cells to insulin reduces, leading to additional problems with calorie intake and weight. By reducing weight the sensitivity to insulin returns to normal. In extreme circumstances, it is this loss of insulin sensitivity that gives rise to late onset diabetes. So there are many good reasons for exercising, not just to burn calories.

AYURVEDIC CONTROL OF BODY WEIGHT

The principle of ayurvedic therapy is to pay attention to balancing the doshas, which constitute who and how you are today on the surface, and to give the correct signals to the intestine. The entire digestive tract is the central control system for our bodies in terms of the food we eat; it even contains the cells that manufacture insulin embedded in the pancreas. If we give it signals that are at odds with reality, it becomes confused and is unable to apply the correct measures to ensure efficient digestion and absorption.

In addition to the exercises mentioned above, you need to stop eating the foods that are on the "No" list in the "Appendix *Kapha*." This is true whatever your basic constitution, except that if you are a pure *vata* person then you will need to balance this with the foods that are recommended on the *vata* list to maintain control of your *vata*. The important rule to remember is never combine foods that fight because they require different types of digestion for a healthy gut.

Also, bear in mind that while high-protein diets are used by some people for weight reduction they are not particularly pleasant, largely because the sweet taste is completely absent from the food. So always have some complex carbohydrate (soluble fiber) in your diet; your large bowel needs it to stay healthy, and keep it separate from the protein. Avoid salty tastes.

Signals to the gut are extremely important. You should avoid ice cold food and drinks at all cost. If the stomach senses "cold" to that degree it will assume that the external weather is cold and react by giving instructions to lay down fat as an insulator against the perceived weather, thus increasing the appetite. We all create this confusion in our intestines every time we eat ice cream in the middle of summer or put ice in our drinks. If you are on a weight-loss program, all drinks should be warm if possible; it does no harm to add an extra bit of "heat" by drinking ginger tea. Just make an infusion of fresh or powdered ginger in some boiling water and drink it regularly. Eat all your food slowly; this will ensure that your mind receives the full taste of the food via the senses. Taste is as important a part of nourishment as the food itself in the ayurvedic system.

If you are a *kapha* or *pitta-kapha* you tend to put on weight by looking at food. There is a good reason for this. When you look at something and crave it, the signal the body receives from the mind tells it to get ready for caloric intake, and existing sugars in the blood stream are converted to storage elements such as glycogen and fat. Then what happens is you feel hungry! So, try to stop looking at or fantasizing about foods you are not going to eat.

How to Eat

In Western society, learning how to eat requires a change in thinking. We are taught to feel guilty about being overweight, but we should try to discard this emotion if we can. Decide from the advice above and the information given under "Balancing the Doshas" which sort of dietary adjustment you are going to make and stick to it, except for one meal a week when you can indulge yourself with whatever you wish. Be assured, this will make almost no difference to the course you have chosen as long as you follow one vitally important rule — do not feel guilty about it. If you do feel guilty, you will come to regard the dietary balance you have chosen as a punishment. It is anything but a punishment and should be enjoyable.

Lastly, be aware of what you are eating at all times. When the feeling of hunger has gone, stop eating. Do not be tempted to clear your plate. We guarantee you will be surprised.

8

OBTAINING AYURVEDIC CARE

It is advisable to obtain advice from an ayurvedic physician to determine the exact nature of your constitution and the degree to which it is presently out of balance, especially if you are suffering overt symptoms of disease. The physician may give you advice on how to change your lifestyle or your diet in order to alleviate your suffering. An added benefit is that the practitioner may detect imbalances you were unaware of, giving you the opportunity to rebalance these aspects *before* they cause a problem.

YOUR FIRST VISIT TO A PRACTITIONER

As with any valid medical system, the first thing that will happen after you have been made comfortable is that a history will be taken. In Western medicine this usually concentrates more on your present circumstances than your past; in Ayurveda it tends to be the other way around. Also, you should expect questions about where you live now, or have lived in the past.

The practitioner will ask you many questions of the sort you have answered in Chapter Five in order to ascertain your *prakruti*. Even if you decide to follow the ayurvedic medical model by visiting a practitioner and not by "doing-it-your-self," you should still go through Chapter Five in detail because many of the questions will be unfamiliar, especially if encountered for the first time in a consulting room. You may also be asked questions about your diet and it is help-ful to take along a list of *exactly* what you have consumed during the previous week. Do this as the week goes by; do not try to do it at the end of the week from memory — it doesn't work.

THE EXAMINATION

Your practitioner will probably make a detailed examination of your tongue. The tongue carries a lot of information about the internal organs of your body and their state of health. It is traditional for a Western medical doctor to ask to see your tongue, but only briefly; the ayurvedic practitioner will study it.

You may be asked for a sample of your urine. If so, it will probably need to be an "early morning" sample that you will have to bring with you on your next visit.

Your practitioner will more than likely take your pulse. In Western medicine this appears to be a fairly straightforward process, but in fact it is quite complex, involving the speed, rhythm, force and shape of what is being felt. Your pulse tells the doctor a lot about your heart, blood vessels and general state of health. Your ayurvedic practitioner will take your pulse from both wrists, probably simultaneously, using three fingers to do it each time; these are placed at the wrist in a special way, as explained earlier. Do not be surprised if your practitioner presses quite firmly with the fingers because it is possible to assess not only your current doshic balance, but also your constitution and the status of the various organs in the body.

You will probably not even notice some of the examinations, especially those required for facial diagnosis, an important part of ayurvedic technique. But you will notice the examination of your nails, at least as important to the ayurvedic practitioner as to your traditional doctor. And you will not miss the fact that your eyes, or more precisely, your irises (the colored part), are being examined, as well as the conjunctiva (the white part).

The Course of Treatment

Your practitioner will explain to you your *prakruti* and what the current state of balance implies, how imbalances are causing the symptoms of disease that have brought you to the consultation, and what to do to set the balance right. Once the course of treatment/lifestyle/diet modification has begun, your practitioner will want to see you again, possibly quite regularly to begin with, to make sure that the doshas are coming back into balance. What is perhaps more important is that the practitioner will be able to advise you in detail about the long-term changes to make in your life to ensure good health in the future.

Other Remedies

Sometimes your physician may recommend certain special ayurvedic treatments, some of which are described briefly below.

Medicinal Herbs

There are many medicinal herbs and substances in the ayurvedic pharmacy that may be used by your practitioner to achieve various effects. Some are very effective in creating balance within unbalanced doshas; some are designed to eliminate *ama* that has accumulated in a tissue. Make sure you know which manufacturer has supplied your herbs and that they have been tested for the presence of heavy metals.

SHIRODHARA

To the Western mind, this treatment may seem somewhat bizarre; it involves the continuous flow of warm oil over the forehead. Strange though it may sound, it is extremely relaxing and may dissolve deep-seated emotional stress. It is sometimes used as part of a more comprehensive treatment known as *panchakarma*.

PANCHAKARMA

This is not a treatment for the faint-hearted. It involves several days of preparation of the body with various forms of deep massage, using a variety of oils followed by a purgative cleansing of the gut. It is extremely effective in balancing the doshas and eliminating stored *ama*, but can only be carried out by a qualified, experienced ayurvedic physician.

FASTING

This process allows the body to digest and remove its *ama* by itself. It must be undertaken only under the strict supervision of an ayurvedic physician. The exact regimen depends upon your constitution and may involve eating only one food, such as rice. It does not necessarily mean stopping eating or drinking!

SWEATING

The physician may recommend, especially following oil treatments, a period of forced sweating to help eliminate *ama* and excess doshas. The methods are many and varied, but all aim to achieve the same objective.

SOME COMMON REMEDIES

DIZZINESS

Crush an onion and forcibly breathe in the aroma.

HEADACHE

Make a teaspoonful of ginger paste from water and dried powdered ginger. Spread this on the inside of a length of bandage sufficient to cover the forehead. Apply and leave in position for an hour or so. Place 3 drops of warm ghee in each nostril and sniff well to relieve tension. Apply sesame oil (untoasted) and massage into the feet and the scalp. Apply pressure massage to both big toes.

INSOMNIA

Apply sesame oil (untoasted) to feet and scalp and gently massage the center of the forehead before retiring. Drink almond milk, made as follows:

soak 10 almonds in warm water for 1–2 hours, then peel

place in a liquidizer/blender and add:

1 cup cow's milk

2 pinches nutmeg

1 pinch dried ginger

1 tsp ground cardamom

liquidize and drink before retiring

RECEDING GUMS

At night, take a mouthful of warm, untoasted sesame oil, but do not swallow. After 5 minutes, spit it out and massage the gums using the index finger. Use dental floss to clean between the teeth. In the morning, chew a small handful of sesame seeds.

SANSKRIT GLOSSARY

Agni: fire, especially digestive fire

Alochak pitta: type of *pitta* related to vision

Ama: toxic material caused by poor digestion

Amla: sour taste

Ananda: bliss

Apana vata: "downward" moving of the five breaths

Artha: goal of "wealth"

Asana: yoga posture

Asthi: bone

Atman: inner self

Avalambak kapha: type of *kapha* in the chest

Ayurveda: spiritual science of life

Bhakti yoga: yoga of devotion

Bhrajak pitta: type of *pitta* related to the complexion

Bhuta: element

Bodhak kapha: type of *kapha* giving rise to taste

Buddhi: "organ" of discrimination

Chakra: spinal center of energy

Charaka: author of old ayurvedic textbooks

Dharma: goal, ideal, law of one's nature

Dhatu: elemental tissue of the body

Dinacharya: daily regimen

Dosha: fault, primary force in body/mind

Doshic: quality relating to the doshas

Gunas: a principle quality of nature

Kapha: water/earth humor

Kledak kapha: type of *kapha* related to digestion

Mamsa: muscle

Manas: the concept of thought in the mind

Medas: fat tissue

Ojas: finest form of subtle energy/cement

Pachaka pitta: type of *pitta* related to digestion

Panchakarma: cleansing actions of vomiting, enemas, purgation, bleeding and nasal medication

Pitta: biological fire/water humor

Prakruti: primary or basic constitution

Prana: breath of life

Pranayama: alternate nostril breathing exercises

Purusha: the inner self or person

Raga: desire

Rajas: *guna* principle of energy/activity/movement

Rajasic: having the quality of *rajas*

Rakta: blood

Ranjak pitta: type of *pitta* causing the color of the blood

Rasa: a) plasma; b) taste

Sadhak pitta: type of *pitta* related to the brain

Samana vata: equalizing breath

Samkhya: system of Indian philosophy
   (*sat* = "truth"; *khya* = "to know")

Sattva: *guna* of harmony and peace

Sattvic: having the quality of *sattva*

Shukra: reproductive fluids

Sleshak kapha: type of *kapha* lubricating the joints

Sukra: goal of happiness

Sushruta: author of old ayurvedic textbooks

Tamas: *guna* of inertia or mass

Tamasic: having the quality of *tamas*

Tanmantra: five principles of sense giving rise to the elements

Tarpak kapha: type of *kapha* related to the brain and nerves

Tejas: mental fire

Udana vata: "upward" moving breath

Vata: air/ether humor

Vayu: alternative name for *vata*

Vedas: ancient books of knowledge presenting the spiritual science of
   awareness

Vikruti: current state, or deviation from natural state of *prakruti*

Vyana vata: the outward moving of the five *vatas* or breaths

APPENDIX VATA

The diet should include:

◆ 40-50% whole grain foods

◆ 10-20% high quality protein

◆ 20-30% fresh cooked vegetables

◆ 10% or more of fresh fruit

▲ — *Okay very occasionally* • — *Okay in moderation only*

FRUITS

No Dried fruit; apples (raw); cranberries; pears; persimmon; pomegranate; prunes (soaked); quince; watermelon.

Note: *Fruits and fruit juices are best consumed by themselves for all doshas.*

Yes Applesauce; sweet fruits; apricots; avocado; bananas; all berries; cherries; coconut; dates; fresh figs; grapefruit; grapes; kiwi; lemons; limes; mangos; nectarines; oranges; papaya; peaches; pineapples; plums; rhubarb; soursop; strawberries; sweet melons.

VEGETABLES

No *In general, dried, frozen or raw vegetables;* eggplant; beet greens; broccoli; burdock root; cabbage; cauliflower; celery; fresh corn; Jerusalem artichoke; jicama; kale; kohlrabi; leafy greens; lettuce; mushrooms (raw); onions (raw); parsley; peas (raw); peppers; potatoes (white); spaghetti squash; spinach (raw); sprouts (all); tomatoes (raw); turnips; turnip greens.

Yes *In general, most cooked vegetables;* acorn squash; artichoke; asparagus; beets; butternut squash; carrots; cilantro; zucchini; cucumber; daikon radish; fenugreek greens; green beans (well cooked); horseradish; leeks (cooked); mustard greens; okra (cooked); olives (black and green); onion (cooked); parsnip; potato (sweet); pumpkin; radish; rutabaga; scallopini squash; spinach (cooked); summer squash; tomato (cooked); watercress; winter squash.

GRAINS

No Barley; bread (yeast); buckwheat; cold, dry, puffed cereals; corn; granola; millet; oats (dry); oat bran; rice cakes; rye; sago; wheat bran.

Yes Amaranth*; oats (cooked); quinoa; rice (all varieties); sprouted wheat bread; wheat.

ANIMAL FOODS

No Lamb; pork; rabbit; venison.

Yes Beef; buffalo; chicken; duck; eggs (including duck eggs); fish; seafood; shrimp; turkey.

LEGUMES

No   Azuki beans; black beans; black-eyed peas; brown lentils; chick peas (garbanzos); dried peas; kidney beans; lima beans; navy beans; pinto beans; soy beans; soy flour; soy powder; spilt peas; tempeh; tofu▲; white beans.

Yes   Black lentils; miso•; mung beans; mung dal; red lentils•; soy cheese•; soy milk (liquid)•; soy sauce•; tepary beans; tofu; tur dal.

NUTS

No   *None listed.*

Yes   Almonds; black walnuts; brazil nuts; cashews; coconut; English walnuts; filberts; hazelnuts; macadamia nuts; peanuts•; pecans; pine nuts; pistachios; walnuts.

SEEDS

No   Psyllium▲; popcorn.

Yes   Chia; flax; pumpkin; sesame; sunflower.

CONDIMENTS

No   Chili pepper▲; ginger (dry); ketchup▲; onion (raw).

Yes   Black pepper•; black sesame seeds; chutney; coconut; coriander leaves•; cottage cheese; grated cheese; daikon radish; dulse; fresh ginger; garlic; ghee; gomasio; hijiki; horseradish; kelp; kombu; lemon; lime; mango chutney; mayonnaise; mint leaves; mustard; onion (cooked); papaya chutney; pickles; salt; seaweed (wet).

SWEETENERS

No   White sugar; maple syrup▲.

Yes Barley malt syrup; brown rice syrup; fructose; fruit juice (concentrated); honey; jaggery; molasses; natural sugar•; sugar cane juice.

DAIRY

No Cow's milk (powder); goat's milk (powder); hard cheese▲; yogurt.

Yes *All okay in moderation:* butter; buttermilk; cow's milk; cottage cheese; goat's milk; goat's cheese; ice cream•; soft cheese; sour cream•.

OILS

No Flax seed.

Yes *All oils okay, especially:* olive; sesame. *External use only:* coconut.

SPICES

No Caraway.

Yes Ajwan; allspice; almond extract; amchoor; anise; asafoetida; basil; bay leaf; black pepper; cardamom; cayenne•; cloves; coriander; cumin; dill; fennel; fenugreek•; garlic; ginger; horseradish; mace; marjoram; mint; mustard seeds; nutmeg; onion (cooked); orange peel; oregano; paprika; parsley; peppermint; pippali; poppy seeds; rosemary; rose water; saffron; sage; savory; spearmint; star anise; tamarind; tarragon; thyme; turmeric; vanilla; wintergreen.

BEVERAGES

No Apple juice; carob▲; carbonated drinks; chocolate; coffee; cold milk drinks; cranberry juice; fig shake; ice cold drinks; pear juice; pungent teas; prune juice▲; tea (black); tomato juice; V-8 juice; **Herb teas:** alfalfa▲; barley▲; blackberry; borage▲; burdock;

chrysanthemum▲; cornsilk; dandelion; ginseng; hibiscus; hops▲; hyssop▲; jasmine▲; mormon tea; nettle▲; passion flower▲; red clover▲; red zinger; sage; strawberry▲; violet▲; wintergreen▲; yarrow; yerba mate▲.

Yes   Alcohol•; almond drink; aloe vera juice; apricot juice; banana shake; berry juice; carrot juice; carrot/ginger juice; cherry juice; cider; coconut milk; hot dairy drinks; grape juice; grapefruit juice; lemonade; mango juice; miso broth; mixed vegetable juice; hot spiced milk; orange juice; papaya juice; peach nectar; pineapple juice; sour juices and teas; soy milk (well spiced and hot); **Grain teas:** Roma; Pero; **Herb teas:** ajwan; bansha (with milk sweetener); basil•; catnip•; chamomile; cinnamon•; clove; comfrey; elderflower; eucalyptus; fennel; fenugreek; ginger (fresh); hawthorn; juniper berry; lavender; lemon balm; lemon grass; licorice; lotus; marshmallow; oat straw; orange peel; osha; pennyroyal; peppermint; raspberry•; rose flower; rose hip; saffron; sarsaparilla; sassafras; spearmint; wild ginger.

OTHER

No   *None listed.*

Yes   Spirulina and other blue-green algae.

APPENDIX *PITTA*

The diet should include:

◆ 40-50% whole grain foods

◆ 15-20% high quality protein

◆ 30-40% fresh cooked vegetables

◆ 15% or more of fresh fruit

▲ — *Okay very occasionally* • — *Okay in moderation only*

FRUITS

No *When any of the following are sour they should not be eaten;* apples; apricots; bananas; berries; cherries; cranberries; grapefruit; green grapes; kiwi▲; lemons; oranges; papaya▲; peaches; pineapples; persimmon; plums; rhubarb; soursop; strawberries; tamarind.

Yes *When the following are sweet they are okay to eat;* apples; apricots; avocado; berries; cherries; coconut;

dates; figs; limes•; mango; melons; oranges; pineapples; plums; pears; pomegranate; prunes; quince; raisins; red grapes; watermelon.

VEGETABLES

No   Eggplant▴; beet greens; beets (raw); carrots (raw); daikon radish; fresh corn; fenugreek greens; garlic; green olives; horseradish; kohlrabi▴; leeks (raw); mustard greens; onions (raw); peppers (hot); radish; spinach (raw); tomatoes; turnips; turnip greens.

Yes   Acorn squash; artichoke; asparagus; beets (cooked); broccoli; Brussels sprouts; burdock root; butternut squash; cabbage; bell pepper; carrots (cooked); cauliflower; zucchini; cucumber; celery; cilantro; fennel; green beans; green peppers; Jerusalem artichoke; jicama; kale; leafy greens; leeks (cooked); lettuce; mushrooms; okra; olives (black); onions (cooked); parsley; parsnip; peas; pumpkin (cooked); rutabaga; spaghetti squash; spinach (cooked); summer squash; sweet potatoes; watercress•; white potatoes; winter squash.

GRAINS

No   Buckwheat; corn; millet; oats (dry); oat granola; quinoa; rice (brown)▴; rye.

Yes   Amaranth; barley; couscous; oat bran•; oats (cooked); rice (basmati); rice cakes; rice (white); wheat; wheat bran; wheat granola.

ANIMAL FOOD

No   Beef; duck; egg yolk; lamb; pork; salmon; seafood.

Yes   Buffalo; egg white; freshwater fish (including shrimp•); rabbit; venison; white chicken; white turkey.

LEGUMES

No Black lentils; tur dal; urad dal.

Yes Azuki beans; black beans; black-eyed peas; chana dal; chick peas (garbanzos); kidney beans; lentils (red and brown); lima beans; mung beans; navy beans; pinto beans; soy beans; soy products: soy cheese; soy flour•; soy milk (liquid); soy powder•; split peas; tempeh; tepary beans; tofu; white beans.

NUTS

No Almonds (plus skin); black walnuts; Brazil nuts; cashews; English walnuts; filberts; hazelnuts; macadamia nuts; peanuts; pecans; pine nuts; pistachios.

Yes Almonds (soaked and peeled); coconut.

SEEDS

No Chia; sesame.

Yes Flax; psyllium; pumpkin•; sunflower.

CONDIMENTS

No Black sesame seeds; chili peppers; daikon radish; garlic; ginger; gomasio; grated cheese; horseradish; kelp; ketchup; mustard; lemon; lime; lime pickle; mango pickle; mayonnaise; onion (raw); papaya chutney; pickles; radish; salt▲; seaweed (unrinsed)▲; sesame seeds; soy sauce; tamarind▲; yogurt (undiluted).

Yes Black pepper•; coconut; coriander leaves; cottage cheese; dulse (well-rinsed)•; ghee; hijiki (well-rinsed)•; kombu•; lettuce; mango chutney; mint leaves.

SWEETENERS

No Honey; jaggery; molasses.

Yes   Barley malt syrup; brown rice syrup; fruit juice (concentrate); fructose; maple syrup; natural sugar; sugar cane juice; white sugar•.

Dairy

No   Buttermilk; feta cheese; hard cheese; salted butter; sour cream; yogurt.

Yes   Cottage cheese; dilute yogurt (1:2-3 pts water); mild soft cheese; ghee; cow's milk; goat's milk; ice cream; unsalted butter.

Oils

No   Almond; apricot; corn; safflower; sesame.

Yes   *In moderation:* flax seed; olive; sunflower; sesame; soy; walnut.

Spices

No   Ajwan; allspice; almond extract; amchoor; anise; asafoetida; basil; bay leaf; caraway▲; cayenne; cloves; dry ginger; fenugreek; garlic (raw); horseradish; mace; marjoram; mustard seeds; nutmeg; onion (raw); oregano; paprika; pippali; poppy seeds; rosemary; sage; savory; star anise; tamarind; tarragon; thyme.

Yes   Basil leaves; black pepper•; cardamom•; cinnamon; coriander; cumin; dill; fennel; fresh ginger; mint; neem leaves•; orange peel•; parsley•; peppermint; rose water; saffron; spearmint; turmeric; vanilla•; wintergreen.

Beverages

No   Alcohol (spirits/wine); banana shake; berry juice (sour); carbonated drinks; cherry juice (sour); coffee; carrot juice; carrot/ginger juice; carrot/vegetable; chocolate; cranberry juice; grapefruit; highly salted drinks; ice cold drinks; lemonade; orange juice▲; miso broth▲; papaya juice; pineapple juice; pungent teas; sour juices and teas; tomato juice; V-8 Juice; **Herb teas:** Ajwan; basil▲; cinnamon▲; cloves; dry ginger; eucalyptus; fenugreek; ginseng; hawthorn; hyssop; juniper berry; Mormon tea; osha; pennyroyal; red zinger; rosehip; sage; sassafras; wild ginger; yerba mate.

Yes Alcohol (beer)•; almond drink; aloe vera juice; apple juice; apricot juice; berry juice (sweet); carob; cherry juice (sweet); coconut milk; cool dairy drinks; date shake; fig shake; goat's milk; grape juice; mango juice; mixed vegetable juice; peach nectar; pear juice; pomegranate juice; prune juice; soy milk; vegetable bouillon; **Grain teas:** Roma; Pero; **Herb teas:** alfalfa; bansha; blackberry; barley; borage; burdock; catnip; chamomile; chicory; chrysanthemum; comfrey; cornsilk; dandelion; elderflower; fennel; fresh ginger; hibiscus; hops; jasmine; lavender; lemon balm; lemon grass; licorice; lotus; marshmallow; nettle; oat straw; orange peel•; passion flower; peppermint; raspberry; red clover; rose flower; saffron; sarsaparilla; spearmint; strawberry; violet; wintergreen; yarrow.

OTHER

No Spirulina and other blue-green algae.

Yes *None listed.*

APPENDIX KAPHA

The diet should include:

◆ 30-40% whole grain foods

◆ 20% high quality protein

◆ 40-50% fresh cooked vegetables

◆ 10% or more of fresh fruit

▲ — *Okay very occasionally* • — *Okay in moderation only*

FRUITS

No   Avocado; bananas: coconut; dates; fresh figs; grape-fruit; grapes▲; kiwi; lemons▲; limes▲; mangoes▲; melons; oranges; papaya; pineapples; plums; rhubarb; soursop; tamarind; watermelon.

Yes   Apples: apple sauce; apricots; berries; cherries; cranberries; dry figs•; peaches; pears; persimmon; pomegranate; prunes; quince; raisins; strawberries•.

VEGETABLES

No Acorn squash; butternut squash; zucchini; cucumber; olives; parsnip▲; pumpkin; raw tomatoes; spaghetti squash▲; sweet potatoes; taro root; winter squash.

Yes *Steamed, raw, pungent and bitter vegetables;* artichoke; asparagus; eggplant; beets; beet greens; bell pepper; broccoli; Brussels sprouts; burdock root; cabbage; carrots; cauliflower; celery; daikon radish; dandelion greens; fennel; fenugreek greens; garlic; green beans; green chilies; horseradish; Jerusalem artichoke; jicama; kale; kohlrabi; kale; leeks; lettuce; mushrooms; mustard greens; okra; onions; parsley; peas; radish; spinach; summer squash; rutabaga; sweetcorn; sweet, hot peppers; turnips; turnip greens; yellow crickneck squash; watercress; white potatoes.

GRAINS

No Brown rice; oats (cooked); quinoa▲; rice cakes▲; spelt▲; wheat; white rice.

Yes Amaranth•; barley; basmati rice (with clove or peppercorns)•; buckwheat; corn; couscous; granola (low-fat); millet oats (dry); oat bran; polenta; rye; wheat bran; sago; sprouted wheat bread (essene); tapioca.

ANIMAL FOODS

No Beef; buffalo; duck; lamb; pork; salmon; sea fish; seafood; tuna.

Yes Chicken eggs (not fried or scrambled with fat); freshwater fish; turkey; rabbit; shrimp; venison.

LEGUMES

No Black lentils; cold tofu; common lentils; soy beans; cold soy milk; kidney beans; mung beans▲; soy cheese; soy flour; soy powder; tempeh.

Yes Azuki beans; black beans; black-eyed peas; chana dal; chick peas (garbanzos); hot tofu•; kala chana; lima beans; navy beans; pinto beans; red/brown lentils; soy milk; soy sausages; split peas; tempeh; tepary beans; tur dal; white beans.

Nuts

No Almond (soaked/peeled)▲; black walnuts; Brazil nuts; cashews; coconut; English walnut; filberts; hazelnuts; macadamia nuts; peanuts; pecans; pine nuts; pistachios.

Yes *None listed.*

Seeds

No Psyllium▲; sesame.

Yes Chia; flax•; popcorn (no salt, no butter); pumpkin•; sunflower•.

Condiments

No Black sesame seeds; cottage cheese; grated cheese; hijiki▲; kelp; ketchup▲; kombu; lemon▲; lime; lime pickle; mango chutney; mango pickles; mayonnaise; papaya chutney; pickles; salt; seaweed▲; sesame seeds; soy sauce; tamarind; vinegar; yogurt.

Yes Black pepper; chili pepper; coriander leaves; daikon radish; dry ginger; dulse (well-rinsed)•; garlic; ghee; horseradish; lettuce; mint leaves; mustard; onions; radish.

Sweeteners

No Barley malt syrup; brown rice syrup; fructose; jaggery; maple syrup; molasses; natural sugar; sugar cane juice; white sugar.

Yes Raw honey•; fruit juice (concentrate).

DAIRY

No Butter (salted); butter (unsalted)▲; buttermilk; cheese of all kinds (except goat); cow's milk; ice cream; sour cream; yogurt (undiluted).

Yes Cottage cheese (from skimmed goat's milk); ghee•; goat's milk; dilute yogurt (1:4 pts water); goat's cheese (not aged and unsalted).

OILS

No Avocado; apricot; coconut; flax seed▲; olive; primrose; safflower; sesame (internally); soy; walnut.

Yes Almond•; corn•; sunflower•.

SPICES

No *None listed.*

Yes Ajwan; allspice; almond extract; anise; asafoetida; basil; bay leaf; black pepper; caraway; cardamom; cayenne; cinnamon; cloves; coriander; cumin; dill; dry ginger; fennel•; fenugreek; garlic; horseradish; mace; mango chutney; marjoram; mint; mustard seeds; neem leaves; nutmeg; onion; orange peel; oregano; paprika; parsley; peppermint; pippali; poppy seeds; rosemary; rose water; saffron; sage; savory; spearmint; sprouts; star anise; tarragon; thyme; turmeric; vanilla•; wintergreen.

BEVERAGES

No Alcohol (beer, spirits and sweet wines); almond drink; banana shake; carbonated drinks; cold dairy drinks; coconut milk; coffee▲; chocolate; date shake; grapefruit juice; highly salted drinks; ice cold drinks; lemonade; miso broth; orange juice; papaya juice; pineapple juice▲; rice milk; sour juices and teas; soy milk (cold); tomato juice; V-8 juice; **Herb teas:** comfrey; lotus; marshmallow; oat straw; Red Zinger; rosehip▲.

Yes   Alcohol, dry (red or white); aloe vera juice; apple juice•; apricot
juice; berry juice; black tea; carob; carrot juice; carrot-ginger
juice; carrot juice combinations; cherry juice (sweet); cranberry
juice; fig shake; hot spiced goat's milk•; grape juice; mango
juice; mixed vegetable juice; peach nectar; pear juice; pomegranate juice; pungent teas; prune juice; soy milk (well-spiced
and warm); **Grain teas:** Cafix; **Herb teas:** ajwan; alfalfa; barley;
basil; bansha; blackberry; borage; burdock; catnip; chamomile;
chicory; chrysanthemum; cinnamon; cloves; corn silk; dandelion; dry ginger; elderflower; eucalyptus; fennel•; fenugreek;
ginseng•; hawthorn; hibiscus; hops; hyssop; jasmine; juniper
berries; lavender; lemon balm; lemon grass; licorice•; Mormon
tea; nettle; orange peel; osha; passion flower; pennyroyal; peppermint; raspberry; red clover; rose flower; saffron; sage; sarsa-
parilla•; sassafras; spearmint; strawberry; violet; wild ginger;
wintergreen; yarrow; yerba mate.

OTHER

No   Potassium salts.

Yes   Brewer's yeast; spirulina and other blue-green algae.

HERBS AND SPICES
TO ASSIST IN
BALANCING THE DOSHAS

Below is a table of common herbs and spices used in cooking, and their properties in terms of their effect upon *vata, pitta* and *kapha*. Use them to modify the effects of the foods you are preparing in the direction indicated in the table.

"+" indicates that it aggravates the dosha

"-" indicates that it reduces or pacifies the dosha

"±" indicates no effect one way or the other

Herb/spice	*Vata*	*Pitta*	*Kapha*
Alfalfa	-	±	-
Aloe Vera	-	-	-
Cardamom	-	+ (in excess)	-
Cayenne pepper	-	+	-
Cinnamon	-	- (small amounts)	-
Cloves	-	+	-
Coriander	-	-	-
Cumin	±	-	-
Garlic	-	+	-
Ghee	-	-	-
Ginger	-	+	-
Honey (uncooked)	-	±	-
Licorice	±	-	±
Mustard	-	+	-
Nutmeg	-	- (small amounts)	-
Pepper	-	+	-
Salt	±	+	+
Turmeric	- (small amounts)	- (small amounts)	-

HELPFUL ADDRESSES

American Holistic Medical Association
4101 Lake Boone Trail, Suite 201
Raleigh, NC 27607

The Ayurvedic Institute
11311 Menaul NE, Suite A
Albuquerque, NM 87112
Tel.: 505 291-9698
Fax: 505-294-7572

National Institute of Ayurvedic Medicine (NIAM)
584 Milltown Road
Brewster, NY 10509
Tel.: 888-246-6426
Tel./fax: 914-278-8700
www.niam.com

RECOMMENDED
READING

Bhagwan Dash, Vaidya, *A Handbook of Ayurveda*, New Delhi, India: 1983.

Frawley, David, *Ayurvedic Healing: A Comprehensive Guide*, Salt Lake City: Passage Press, 1992.

Heyn, Birgit, *Ayurvedic Medicine: The Gentle Strength of Indian Healing*, Wellingborough: Thorsons, 1987.

Lad, Usha and Lad, Vasant, *Ayurvedic Cooking for Self-Healing*, Albuquerque: The Ayurvedic Press, 1994.

Lad, Vasant, *Ayurveda: The Science of Self-Healing*, Sante Fe: Lotus Press, 1984.

Lad, Vasant and Frawley, David, *The Yoga of Herbs*, Sante Fe: Lotus Press, 1986.

Murthy, K. R. Sikantha (tr.), *Astanga Hrdayam* (Vols. 1, 2 and 3), Varanasi, India: 1992.

Ranade, Subhash, *Natural Healing Through Ayurveda*, Salt Lake City: Passage Press, 1993.

Svoboda, Robert, *Ayurveda: Life, Health and Longevity*, London: Arkana, 1992

Svoboda, Robert, *Prakruti: Your Ayurvedic Constitution*, Albuquerque: Geocom, 1988.

INDEX

ULYSSES PRESS HEALTH BOOKS

DISCOVER HANDBOOKS

Easy to follow and authoritative, *Discover Handbooks* reveal an array of alternative therapies from around the world and demonstrate how to incorporate them into a program of good health.

Each book opens with information on the history and principles of the particular technique, then presents practical and straightforward guidance on ways in which it can be applied. Offering the tools needed to achieve and maintain an optimal state of health, the approach is one of personal improvement and self-reliance. Each of the books features: an introduction to the discipline; an explanation of its philosophy; step-by-step guide to its implementation; clear diagrams and charts; and case studies.

DISCOVER AYURVEDA
ISBN 1-56975-081-5, 128 pp, $8.95

DISCOVER COLOR THERAPY
ISBN 1-56975-093-9, 144 pp, $8.95

DISCOVER ESSENTIAL OILS
ISBN 1-56975-080-7, 128 pp, $8.95

DISCOVER FLOWER ESSENCES
ISBN 1-56975-099-8, 120 pp, $8.95

DISCOVER MEDITATION
ISBN 1-56975-113-7, 144 pp, $8.95

DISCOVER NUTRITIONAL THERAPY
ISBN 1-56975-135-8, 120 pp, $8.95

DISCOVER OSTEOPATHY
ISBN 1-56975-115-3, 132 pp, $8.95

DISCOVER REFLEXOLOGY
ISBN 1-56975-112-9, 132 pp, $8.95

DISCOVER SHIATSU
ISBN 1-56975-082-3, 128 pp, $8.95

A NATURAL APPROACH BOOKS

Written in a friendly, nontechnical style, *A Natural Approach* books address specific health issues and show you how to take an active part in your own treatment. Whether you suffer from panic attacks, endometriosis or depression, each book will provide you with a thorough understanding of your condition and detail organic solutions that offer immediate relief for your symptoms and effectively remedy their underlying causes.

Believing that disease is more than a combination of symptoms, these books offer integrated mind/body programs that take a positive, preventative approach. Since traditional drug therapy is not always the best solution (and can sometimes be the problem), these guides show how to use alternative treatments to supplement or replace conventional medicine.

ANXIETY & DEPRESSION
ISBN 1-56975-118-8, 144 pp, $9.95

IRRITABLE BOWEL SYNDROME
ISBN 1-56975-030-0, 240 pp, $11.95

ENDOMETRIOSIS
ISBN 1-56975-088-2, 120 pp, $8.95

MIGRAINES
ISBN 1-56975-140-4, 156 pp, $8.95

FREE YOURSELF FROM TRANQUILIZERS & SLEEPING PILLS
ISBN 1-56975-074-2, 192 pp, $9.95

PANIC ATTACKS
ISBN 1-56975-045-9, 148 pp, $8.95

IRRITABLE BLADDER & INCONTINENCE
ISBN 1-56975-089-0, 108 pp, $8.95

THE NATURAL HEALER BOOKS

As home remedies and alternative treatments become increasingly accepted into the medical mainstream, people want information—not just hype and unproven claims—about the remedies they see in health food stores. *The Natural Healer* books detail how these natural remedies have been used throughout history and how to safely incorporate them into an overall plan for maintaining good health.

CIDER VINEGAR
ISBN 1-56975-141-2, 120 pp, $8.95

GARLIC
ISBN 1-56975-097-1, 120 pp, $8.95

THE ANCIENT AND
HEALING ARTS BOOKS

The Ancient and Healing Arts books recount the development of healing art forms that have been used for thousands of years. Beautifully illustrated with full color on every page, they discuss the benefits of these time-honored techniques and offer detailed instructions on their use.

THE ANCIENT AND HEALING ART OF
AROMATHERAPY
ISBN 1-56975-094-7, 96 pp, $14.95

THE ANCIENT AND HEALING ART OF
CHINESE HERBALISM
ISBN 1-56975-139-0, 96 pp, $14.95

OTHER HEALTH TITLES

THE BOOK OF KOMBUCHA
ISBN 1-56975-049-1, 160 pp, $11.95
Explains the benefits of and addresses concerns about Kombucha, the widely used Chinese "tea mushroom."

HEPATITIS C: A PERSONAL GUIDE TO GOOD HEALTH
ISBN 1-56975-091-2, 172 pp, $12.95
Identifies the causes and symptoms of hepatitis C and presents conventional and alternative treatments for coping with the disease.

KNOW YOUR BODY: THE ATLAS OF ANATOMY
ISBN 1-56975-021-1, 160 pp, $12.95
Presents a full-color guide to the structure of the human body.

MOOD FOODS
ISBN 1-56975-023-8, 192 pp, $9.95
Shows how the foods you eat influence your emotions and behavior.

YOUR NATURAL PREGNANCY: A GUIDE TO COMPLEMENTARY THERAPIES
ISBN 1-56975-059-9, 240 pp, $16.95
Details alternative therapies ranging from aromatherapy to yoga that can benefit pregnant women.

To order these books call 800-377-2542, fax 510-601-8307 or write to Ulysses Press, P.O. Box 3440, Berkeley, CA 94703-3440. All retail orders are shipped free of charge. California residents must include sales tax. Allow two to three weeks for delivery.

Angela Hope-Murray studied at the Ayurveda Wellness Center in the United States and practices Ayurveda in the U.K. Tony Pickup is a physician and consultant to pharmaceutical and health food industries.